THE WATER METABOLISM OF THE FETUS

CONTRIBUTORS

ALLAN C. BARNES

Vice-President
The Rockefeller Foundation
New York, New York
Formerly Professor and Chairman
Department of Gynecology and Obstetrics
The Johns Hopkins University School of Medicine
Baltimore, Maryland

JOHN D. BIGGERS

Professor of Population Dynamics
The Johns Hopkins University School of Hygiene
Associate Professor
Department of Gynecology and Obstetrics
The Johns Hopkins University School of Medicine
Baltimore, Maryland

IRVIN M. CUSHNER

Associate Professor
Department of Gynecology and Obstetrics
The Johns Hopkins University School of Medicine
Baltimore, Maryland

CHARLES H. HENDRICKS

Professor and Chairman
Department of Obstetrics and Gynecology
University of North Carolina School of Medicine
Chapel Hill, North Carolina

BRIAN LITTLE

Professor of Obstetrics and Gynecology
Department of Reproductive Biology
Case Western Reserve University School of Medicine
Director, Department of Obstetrics and Gynecology
Cleveland Metropolitan General Hospital
Cleveland, Ohio

HENRY L. NADLER

Chairman of the Department of Pediatrics
Northwestern University Medical School
Head, Division of Genetics
Children's Memorial Hospital
Chicago, Illinois

A. ELMORE SEEDS

Professor
Department of Obstetrics and Gynecology
Georgetown University School of Medicine
Washington, D.C.
Formerly Associate Professor
Department of Gynecology and Obstetrics
The Johns Hopkins University School of Medicine
Baltimore, Maryland

PREFACE

The literature on amniotic fluid, its physiology and its diagnostic uses, has increased tremendously within the past few years. From the simple concept of a "cushion for the baby," knowledge concerning its dynamism has developed to the point where it is recognized that amniotic fluid has a life of its own, intimately related metabolically to that of the fetus and with considerable fetal prognostic significance. The articles on these subjects have appeared in profusion in the last decade and are widely spread throughout the medical journals. At no place, however, are they gathered together and it is to this task that the editors have addressed themselves.

A collation of the current information concerning amniotic fluid has been achieved in this slender volume for the convenience of the physician to provide in one text the contemporary status of our knowledge of amniotic fluid.

Such an objective could only be approached by asking the true experts in this field each to contribute an appropriate chapter bringing the subject up-to-date. This has been achieved. The editors are primarily grateful to the individual authors whose work has made this publication possible. The reader will quickly agree, we are sure, that they not only write from authority but they present their material exceedingly well.

The editors' role has been to gather and organize; to edit (minimally); and, on occasion, to weave together. One must echo Montaigne's statement, "I have gathered me a bunch of posies in other men's gardens; naught but the string that binds them is mine own."

In addition to the individual authors, we are obligated to Miss Ann Royston for her cheerful assistance in getting the manuscript ready for the publishers.

ALLAN C. BARNES
A. ELMORE SEEDS

CONTENTS

THE WATER METABOLISM OF THE FETUS

Chapter 1

MAMMALIAN BLASTOCYST AND AMNION FORMATION

John D. Biggers

INTRODUCTION

The amnion is one of the extra-embryonic membranes which appears very early in development. The mode of its formation was discussed in 1945, by Arthur T. Hertig, in the eighth Harry Burr Ferris Lecture at Yale University, entirely in terms of the eleven then known early human embryos. His lecture, "On the Development of the Amnion and Exocoelomic Membrane in the Pre-villous Human Ovum," was published in the *Yale Journal of Biology and Medicine.* At the end of his address, Hertig concluded:

> From a series of eleven normal human ova . . . is demonstrated the progressive *in situ* delamination of primitive mesoblast, exocoelomic membrane, and amnion from the trophoblast. . . . The amnion begins to delaminate from adjacent trophoblast during the eighth day and gradually encloses the concave space above the germ-disc during the next five days to form the amniotic cavity.
>
> Observations on two pathological pre-villous human ova deficient in embryonic and trophoblastic tissues, respectively show that the exocoelomic membrane will form in the absence of an embryo, although the amnion will not. . . .

Our knowledge of the nature and mechanism of amnion formation in any mammalian species has not increased very much since Hertig's lecture. However, the amnion is one of the first structures to develop from the blastocyst, and in many species both structures arise by the same process—cavitation. The formation of the

Note—The preparation of this chapter has been made possible by grants from the Ford Foundation, National Institute of Child Health and Human Development and the Population Council.

blastocyst will, therefore, be discussed first. In particular, emphasis will be given to the kinetic aspects involved in the formation of the blastocyst, and its transformation into a structure containing an early embryo within an amniotic cavity.

A BRIEF REVIEW OF EARLY DEVELOPMENT

Students of the general principles which govern animal development recognize a series of early critical processes: fertilization, cleavage, blastula formation, gastrulation, and the formation of the extra-embryonic parts. In mammals, fertilization takes place in the ampullary region of the fallopian tube; the cleavage divisions and blastula formation occur as the embryo journeys down the fallopian tube into the uterus, and gastrulation and formation of the extra-embryonic parts is achieved in the uterus. The blastula is specifically called the *blastocyst;* it is at first free in the uterine lumen, but it eventually adheres to the endometrium, the first phase of implantation.[37] The extra-embryonic parts develop soon afterwards and are, therefore, intimately related in time with implantation and the formation of the placenta. Mossman[36] has presented strong evidence from studies in comparative anatomy to show that the modes of amnion formation and implantation are closely correlated. Nevertheless, the formation of the extra-embryonic parts do not seem to be causally related to the maternal-embryonic interactions involved in implantation. Thus, we will treat the problem of amnion formation entirely as a problem of embryonic development.

No attempt will be made to cover all the literature. The early development of mammals is described in many places. An excellent account of the processes involved, compared with analogous processes in nonmammalian forms, is given by Balinsky,[1] and his terminology is adopted in this chapter. A thorough coverage of many aspects of the mammalian blastocyst is found in Blandau.[2] The classical morphological literature provides extensive descriptions of the formation of the amnion in many species of mammals; those interested should refer to Hubrecht,[27] Da Costa,[9] Mossman,[36] and Boyd and Hamilton.[4]

BLASTOCYST

Structure

In mammals, the fertilized ovum undergoes a series of mitotic divisions to form a ball of cells called the *morula.* Soon afterwards, the embryo develops into the blastocyst—a hollow, fluid-filled structure. All blastocysts have some general characteristics (Fig. 1-1). Most of the wall of the blastocyst is only one cell thick. This thickening may be flat as in the rabbit and many rodents, or rather pendulous so that it protrudes into the central cavity, as in some carnivores. The point marking the center of the thickened area on the surface of the blastocysts is called the *embryonic pole,* and the opposite point is the *abembryonic pole.* The cells of the blastocyst are arranged geometrically so that asymmetry exists on either side of planes at right angles to the axis joining the embryonic and abembryonic poles of the embryo, while symmetry exists on either side of all planes through the polar axis.

The formation of the mammalian blastocyst is one of the first obvious morphological manifestations of regionalization—one of several basic processes of embryological development.[52] By this

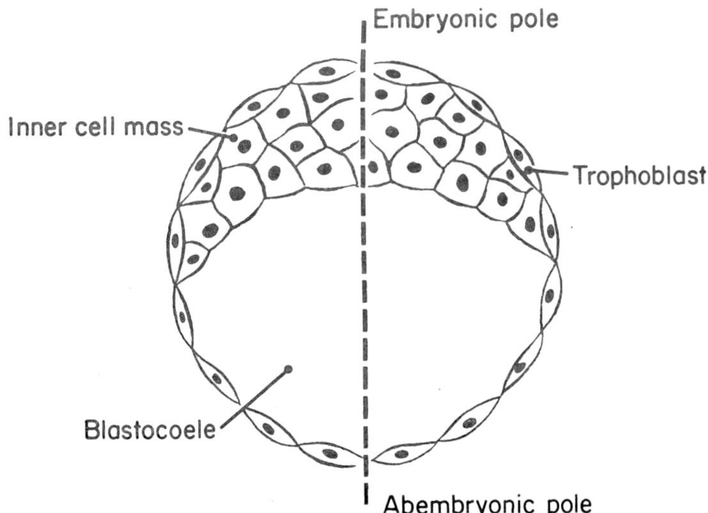

FIGURE 1-1. The parts of a typical blastocyst.

stage of development two major cellular assemblies can already be recognized—the *trophoblast* and the *inner cell mass.* Let us be precise in the meaning of these two terms. Histochemical studies on the rat show that the blastocyst is entirely enveloped by a single layer of cells which appears pale when stained with basic dyes such as toluidine blue and which stains negatively for alkaline phosphatase.[14] In contrast, the aggregate of cells inside the blastocyst stains strongly with toluidine blue and gives a positive alkaline phosphatase reaction. The enveloping cells are called the *trophoblast* and the internal mass the *inner cell mass.* The internal fluid-filled cavity is called the *blastocoele.*

Growth

Since considerable variation occurs between species, two extreme types of development will be examined. At one extreme are the mouse, rat, hamster, and guinea pig blastocysts which implant when their size is only slightly larger than the tubal egg. At the opposite extreme are the rabbit and pig blastocysts which increase in size by several orders of magnitude as soon as they reach the uterus. In order to contrast the two extremes, we will describe the behavior of mouse and rabbit blastocysts in some detail.

The form of the living mouse blastocyst flushed from the uterus at different times after mating has been described by Dickson.[18] The "average" mouse blastocyst obtained from the uterus at noon on the fourth day of pregnancy is spherical and about 96 μm in diameter. It contains a small blastocoele and is still encased in the zona pellucida. At 10:00 P.M. on the fourth day the zona is lost. At 1:00 P.M. on the fifth day the giant-cell transformation starts at the abembryonic pole, and begins to sweep across the blastocyst to the region of the inner cell mass. At the beginning of this process the length of the blastocyst is about 108 μm. By 3:00 A.M. on the fifth day the giant-cell transformation is halfway to the edge of the inner cell mass and the blastocyst is about 151 μm long. By noon on the fifth day the giant-cell transformation is complete and the blastocyst is 186 μm in length. Thus, the blastocyst of the mouse roughly doubles its size during its "free-living" period in the uterus. How much of this is due to cellular growth and how much to an increase in the volume of the blastcoele is unknown.

The behavior of the rabbit blastocyst, however, is very different.[15] Cavity formation can be detected first at 3.5 days after fertilization. Thereafter, the volume of the blastocyst and its surface area rapidly increases (Table 1-I). The change in size seems

TABLE 1-I

THE MEAN VOLUME, MEAN SURFACE AREA AND TOTAL TROPHOBLAST CELL NUMBER OF RABBIT BLASTOCYSTS OF DIFFERENT AGES

Age (days)	*Volume (μl)*	*Surface Area (μm²)†*	*Trophoblast Cell Number*
3	0.002	0.080	—
4	0.0157	0.304	983
5	0.565	2.61	8,930
6	11.5	24.8	80,259
7	66.1	78.9	255,339
8	345	238	770,227

From Daniel.[15]

†Systeme International d'Unites

largely due to the accumulation of fluid in the blastocoele, although this accommodation also involves cell multiplication. These relative quantitative aspects of the growth of the blastocyst have not been thoroughly examined.

THE BLASTOCOELE FLUID

Rate of Formation

Only the rabbit blastocyst has been studied from a biochemical point of view, and this is because of its ready availability and size. Samples of blastocoele fluid can be collected from the fifth day onwards,[21] though most work done prior to this time starts with fluid from the 7-day-old blastocyst. Consequently, the composition of the blastocoele fluid has received considerable attention, and the subject has been thoroughly reviewed recently.[33] We will consider only those biochemical aspects involved in the formation of the blastocoele fluid.

The blastocyst of the rabbit rapidly expands due to the accumulation of fluid in the blastocoele, and this fluid has many substances dissolved in it.[33] Table 1-II shows the concentrations of

TABLE 1-II

CONCENTRATIONS OF POTASSIUM, SODIUM AND CHLORIDE IONS IN 6- TO 8-DAY-OLD RABBIT BLASTOCOELE FLUID

	Concentration (mEq/l)			
Age (days)	*K^+*	*Na^+*	*Cl^-*	*Reference*
6	9.2	144	88	Smith[42]
7	12	122	73	Lutwak-Mann[31]
8	5.5	137	83.5	Lutwak-Mann[31]

sodium, potassium, and chloride in the blastocoele fluid of 6- to 8-day-old rabbit blastocysts. The mere presence of these ions in the blastocoele fluid means they also must have been accumulated during its formation.

A better appreciation of the mechanisms involved in the formation of blastocoele fluid is gained if the process is described in kinetic terms. For a given stage of development (t) let

dV/dt = rate of accumulation of the blastocoele fluid, and

C_{ion} = the instantaneous concentration of an ion in the blastocoele fluid being formed.

Over a short interval, let us assume as a first approximation that an estimate of C_{ion} is given by the concentration of the ion in the fluid present in the blastocoele. This assumption is reasonable if the concentration of the ion in the blastocoele fluid is not rapidly changing. It then follows that the net rate of accumulation of the ion at time t is given by

$$dA/dt = C_{ion}\ dV/dt.$$

Sufficient data are present in the literature for such estimates of dA/dt to be made, and the results are shown in Table 1-III. The

TABLE 1-III

RATE OF ACCUMULATION OF BLASTOCOELE FLUID AND THE IONS (dAion/dt): POTASSIUM, SODIUM AND CHLORIDE IN RABBIT EMBRYOS OF VARIOUS AGES

Age (days)	*Blastocoele fluid*		*dAion/dt (mEq/hr)*		
	dV/dt (1/hr)	*per cell (pl/hr)*	K^+	Na^+	Cl^-
4	0.0023	2.29	—	—	—
5	0.068	7.61	—	—	—
6	0.8	9.96	7.36	115.2	70.4
7	5.6	22.0	67.2	683	409
8	18.0	23.4	99	2,466	1,503

From Daniel.[15]

calculations clearly show that large amounts of K^+, Na^+ and Cl^- are accumulated in the blastocoele fluid. Moreover, a comparison of the rates of accumulation of Na^+ and Cl^- on days 6 and 8 of development show the uptake of both increases about 21 times. In contrast the rate of accumulation of K^+ increases only about 13 times.

There is little doubt that the water and various ions that accumulate in the blastocoele are derived from outside of the blastocyst. Prior to the seventh day of development the source is the uterine fluid, and from 7 days onward the source is from the maternal plasma.

Cellular Wall

The wall of the blastocyst is a living membrane across which occurs the transfer of materials. Let us look at its structure in the rat as described by Schlafke and Enders.[40]

> A distinct junctional complex is invariably present at the apical end of the lateral cell boundaries of the trophoblast cells. This complex consists of a region of close opposition and possible fusion of the cell membranes surrounded by a slightly dense zone of cytoplasm. Within the complex, areas where the membranes diverge may also be found.

> . . . The cell borders are relatively straight below the junctional complex. However, towards the basal end a few microvilli either interdigitate between the cells or project into the cavity of the blastocyst.

The appearance of similar junctions have also been described in the mouse.[6] The transport of ions into the blastocyst is, therefore, across a membrane composed of cells linked by close junctional complexes.

The permanence of this cellular barrier is of some interest since studies on blastocysts *in vitro*, using time-lapse cinematography, have shown that the blastocyst undergoes rhythmic cycles of contraction and expansion. The phenomenon was first seen in the rabbit by Lewis and Gregory,[30] and then in the mouse by Kuhl and Friedrich-Freska[29] and Kuhl.[28] Since then it has been studied in the mouse by Borghese and Cassini,[3] Cole and Paul[7] and Mulnard.[39] The changes involve considerable alterations in volume (Fig. 1-2), and loss of nearly half of the blastocoele fluid. The loss is fairly rapid, as though the blastocyst suddenly becomes leaky. The loss of fluid may possibly be associated with a change in the properties of the junctional complexes.

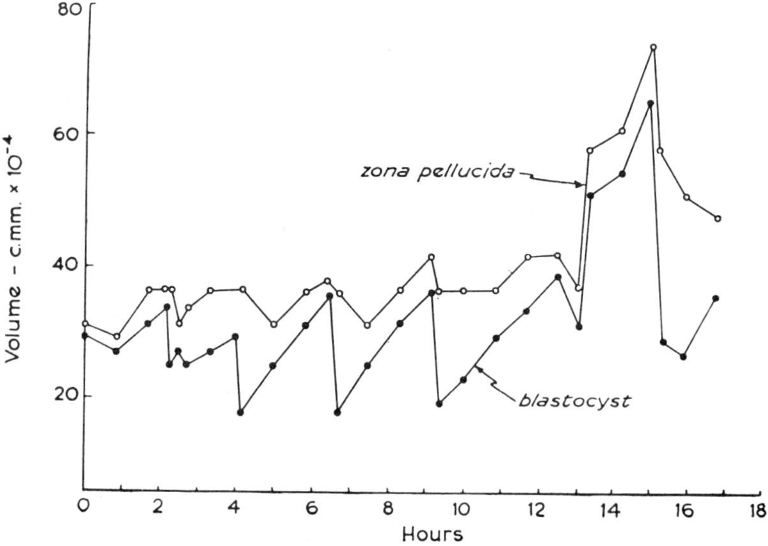

FIGURE 1-2. Volume changes *in vitro* of a mouse blastocyst-measured by frame analysis of a time-lapse film (after Cole and Paul, 1965).

In order to accommodate the blastocoele fluid the number of cells in the trophoblast wall increases by mitosis. The number of cells in the rabbit has been estimated by Daniel[15] and is shown in Table 1-I. Using these estimates of cell number we can calculate the rate of accumulation of blastocoele fluid per trophoblast cell. The results shown in Table 1-III indicate that the ability of the cells to produce blastocoele fluid increases with development.

Transport Across the Trophoblast

6-day-old Rabbit Blastocyst

Active Transport. Studies with radioactive isotopes suggested that active transport of molecules into the blastocoele fluid does occur.[34] Recently, two studies have shown a potential difference across the blastocyst wall of the 5½- and 6-day-old rabbit blastocyst.[11, 21] The observed value varied with the conditions of measurement, but the inside of the blastocyst was negative with respect to the outside. Both Gamow and Daniel[21] and Cross and Brinster[12] have shown that the potential difference vanishes if the blastocysts are exposed to anoxia and such metabolic inhibitors as dinitrophenol, sodium cyanide, and iodoacetic acid, showing that the expenditure of energy is required to maintain the difference.

Cross[10] has demonstrated active transport directly in the 6-day-old rabbit blastocyst. A method has been developed to perfuse the blastocoele with the same fluid that bathes the blastocyst, thereby eliminating concentration gradients across the blastocyst wall. Simultaneously, electrical currents were applied across the blastocyst wall to neutralize the normal potential difference and thereby eliminate electrical gradients. Under these conditions an average short-circuit current of 40 ± 5.2 nA/mm^2, based on 7 observations, could be demonstrated for up to 210 min. The significant short-circuit current reflects the net active transport of ions across the wall of the 6-day-old rabbit blastocyst. Smith[42] has shown that cooling to 0° C and the inhibitor ouabain inhibit the accumulation of fluid and Na^+ and Cl^-.

Chemical Potential of Water. Comparisons have been made in the rabbit between the osmolarity of uterine fluid and the blastocoele fluid on the fifth day of pregnancy.[21, 32, 50] All investigators agree that from the sixth day of pregnancy the osmolarity of uterine fluid is lower than that of the blastocoele fluid.

If we let μu and μb represent the chemical potential of water in the uterine and blastocoele fluids respectively, then the chemical potential gradient across the blastocoele wall ($\Delta\mu$) is given by

$$\Delta\mu = \mu_u - \mu_b = L_f \ (\Delta T_b - \Delta T_u)/273$$

where L_f is the latent heat of fusion, ΔT_u, ΔT_b are the observed depressions of freezing point of uterine and blastocoele fluids respectively, and $\Delta\mu$ is expressed in liter atmospheres per mole. Estimates of $\Delta\mu$ from the data of Lutwak-Mann[32] and Tuft and Boving[50] for the 6-day-old blastocyst give 6.08 and 3.91 ml atmos/ mol^{-1} respectively. The positive sign indicates that water will flow passively along a chemical potential gradient from the uterine fluid into the blastocoele.

Chemical Potential Gradient and Active Transport at Different Stages of Development. The studies reviewed so far provide evidence for active transport of ions, and the passive movement of water across the wall of the 6-day-old rabbit blastocyst.

The chemical potential gradient for water and the potential difference across the blastocyst wall at different stages of development in the rabbit are shown in Figure 1-3. The gradient is not significantly different from zero on the fourth day indicating no passive flow of water across the wall at this time. On the fifth and sixth days, $\Delta\mu$ is positive, indicating that a passive flow of water occurs from the uterine fluid into the blastocyst. On the seventh and eighth days implantation has begun, and any transfer of water is between the maternal blood plasma and the blastocoele. At these stages $\Delta\mu$ is negative, indicating that a passive transfer of water occurs from the blastocoele to the plasma. Thus, on the fourth, seventh and eighth days of development water is transferred into the blastocoele by processes different from passive diffusion. An important question is whether passive diffusion is a significant component in the transfer of water from the uterine

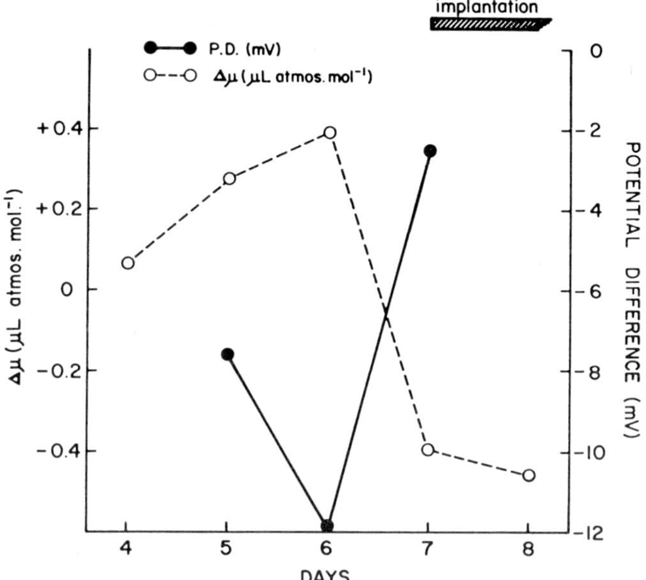

FIGURE 1-3. The chemical potential ($\Delta\mu$) (from Tuft and Boving, 1970) and the potential differences (P.D.) (from Cross and Brinster, 1969) of the blastocoele fluid in rabbit blastocysts 4 to 8 days old.

fluid to the blastocoele on days 5 and 6. There is no quantitative data on this question, but the fact the blastocoele rapidly expands at this time suggests that mechanisms in addition to passive transport are involved. An estimate of the rate that energy is required to move water into the blastocoele of a 7-day-old rabbit embryo is 35μcal/hour^{-1}. Respiration at this stage is provided at a much greater rate – 4.04 mcal/hour.$^{-1}$

The potential difference across the trophoblast is negative on days 5, 6, and 7, suggesting that active transport of ions occurs; however, the unequivocal demonstration of active transport on days 5 and 7 is still required.

The results shown in Figure 1-3 demonstrate a considerable change in events at the time implantation is initiated. Lutwak-Mann[31] pointed out that at 7 days the ionic composition of blastocoele fluid becomes more like that of the maternal plasma.

Future Studies

The evidence that has been reviewed shows that the formation of the blastocoele fluid involves the active transport of ions across the trophoblast wall, together with considerable amounts of water. This information is sufficient to suggest further courses of study. There are two major areas of investigation: first, the analysis of solute and solvent transfer in terms of "macroscopic" physical-chemical theory, and second, a "microscopic" analysis of the cellular mechanisms involved.

Macroscopic Analysis

The limited evidence available on the formation of blastocoele fluid strongly suggests that the process involves irreversible net fluxes of solutes and a solvent—in this case water. Such nonequilibrium processes can be analyzed either by kinetic theory, or Onsager's theory of the thermodynamics of irreversible processes.[17, 43] The classical thermodynamic theory based on functional semipermeable membranes is not appropriate. Recently Tuft and Boving[50] have argued that the flux of water into the blastocoele is active, involving the expenditure of energy. The application of the theory of irreversible processes using the approach of Diamond,[16] in studies on the gallbladder, may help decide the central question as to whether active transport of water occurs in the formation of the blastocoele fluid.

Microscopic Analysis

The thermodynamic methods just described do not contribute to our knowledge of the cellular mechanisms concerned in coupled water and solute fluxes. The principles involved are of general physiological interest, and they have been at the cellular level studied in the passage of water and solutes across the wall of the gallbladder. Two major theories have been put forward: (1) the double membrane theory of Curran[13] and Durbin,[19] and (2) the theory of local osmosis.[16] A detailed discussion of these theories is given by Dick.[17] The relevance of these two theories to the formation of blastocoele fluid has been discussed by Gamow and

Daniel,[21] and they suggest that local osmosis is the mechanism involved. Their conclusion, however, may be premature. First, both theories assume that water is not actively transported, and it has already been shown that this assumption is still unsettled. Furthermore, according to Dick,[17] the main argument for the local osmosis theory is that, "provided solute flow is not too rapid nor the water permeability of the barrier too low to allow osmotic equilibrium, then the solution transferred would always be isosmotic irrespectively of the concentration of the bathing solution." Gamow and Daniel[21] claim that the condition of isosmolarity is fulfilled, but the more extensive evidence of Tuft and Boving[50] indicates this may not be so.

It is clear that future research needs to examine whether the active transport of water is involved in the formation of blastocoele fluid, and also the osmolarity of the fluid transferred. Fortunately, the possibility exists of developing techniques to investigate this problem quantitatively. The problem has inherent physiological interest, but is especially intriguing since it is also one of the earliest functional differentiations in embryonic development.

So far, no attention has been given to the nature of the cells which form the boundary of the blastocoele. Are they homogeneous, or do those adjacent to the inner cell mass differ from the trophoblast? At present we have no information on this point although the fact that cavitation does not occur between the cells of the inner cell mass suggests that the cellular adhesions between them have unique features. The possibility that the cells bounding the blastocoele differ in their ability to transport substances should be kept in mind, since heterogeneity of function in different parts of the lining cells could create important directional fluxes of the constituents of the blastcoele fluid and the external environment (see "Microscopic Analysis" previously discussed).

FORMATION OF THE BLASTOCYST

A blastocyst forms by the accumulation of fluid within a morula. Many morphological studies (for example, Mulnard,[39] in the mouse) have shown that the fluid does not collect in the center of the morula but in an eccentric position. It is this process that creates the asymmetric form of the blastocyst. What factors are involved in the formation of this asymmetric cyst-like structure? It is helpful to initially define some cyst-like structures which form useful models in the analysis of this problem; such structures were originally recognized by Tarkowski and Wróblewska[47] in their work on the development of isolated blastomeres.

1. *Trophoblastic vesicle* (Fig. 1-4a). A structure in which all cells contribute to the wall of the vesicle, and the inner cell mass is absent altogether.

2. *False blastocyst* (Fig. 1-4b). A structure in which all cells participate in forming the wall of the vesicle, but some are thickened in one region giving the impression of an inner cell mass.

3. *Blastocyst* (Fig. 1-4c). A structure with inner cell mass cells covered by trophoblastic cells.

All three structures shown in Figure 1-4 are formed by the accumulation of fluid within a ball of cells. In the case of the trophoblastic vesicle and the false blastocyst this involves at least two phenomena: the creation of boundary conditions within which fluid can accumulate, and the transport of fluid into this bounded space. The simplest of these structures is the trophoblastic vesicle; if we assume all the cells are similar, the formation of the

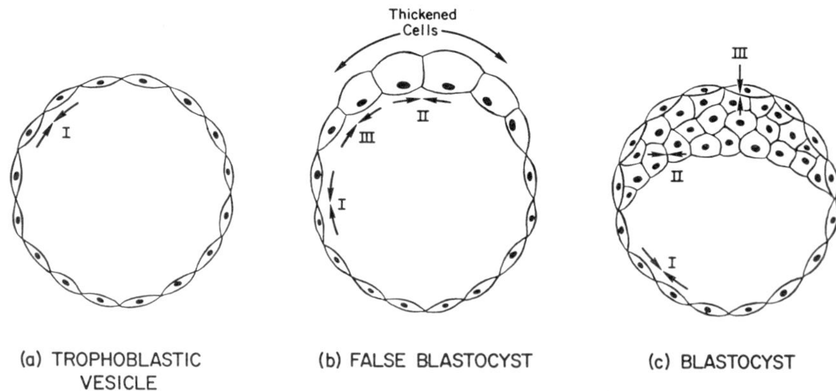

FIGURE 1-4. Schematic diagrams of (a) a trophoblastic vesicle, (b) a false blastocyst, and (c) a normal blastocyst, based on the descriptions of Tarkowski and Wroblewska (1967). The opposing arrows indicate possible sites of specialized cell contacts.

wall merely involves the formation of appropriate junctional complexes between the adjacent cells. The transport of fluid into the cyst will be uniform over the entire surface. The false blastocyst is more complex since a localized region of the wall differentiates it from the rest. Three regions of junctional complex are required for its formation (Fig. 1-4b): I—between cells of the trophoblast, II—between cells in the thickened area, and III—between the cells at the junction of the differentiated areas. This model raises the possibility that the transport of fluid in the two differentiated areas of the wall may differ. The blastocyst is a more complex structure (Fig. 1-4c). It is surrounded by trophoblast cells considered uniform with similar junctional complexes between them (I). Inside is a mass of cells presumably held together by similar junctional complexes (II). This adherent collection of cells is the inner cell mass. The inner cell mass is fixed to the trophoblast in one area, and its position leads to the asymmetry of the blastocyst. Presumably special junctions hold the cells of the inner cell mass to the outer trophoblast wall (III). Occasionally two inner cell masses may be contiguous with different areas of the trophoblast and lead to a form of monozygotic twinning.[8] Thus, the formation of the blastocyst involves the internal differentiation and localization of the inner cell mass, as well as the creation of boundary conditions and the transport of fluid into the bounded space. As in the case of the false blastocyst, there is a real possibility of differential fluid transport through the different parts of the wall.

The three following questions concerning the formation of the blastocyst will now be discussed:

1. How are the boundary conditions created?
2. When does a blastocoele start to form?
3. How does the blastocoele develop in an eccentric position?

How Are the Boundary Conditions of the Blastocoele Created?

The blastocoele is bounded by cells and the junctions between them. Thus, the properties of the boundary layer are determined by the permeability characteristics of the cells and the tightness of the cell junctions binding the cells together. It has already been suggested that the boundary is a layer of cells capable of transferring materials into the blastocyst by energy-dependent coupled solute and water fluxes.

The nature of the contacts between the cells of the early rat embryo have been described by Schlafke and Enders[40] and Enders.[20] At the 4-cell stage the blastomeres are closely apposed, and have numerous regions where the adjacent membranes are 20 to 30 nm apart. By the 8-cell stage junctional complexes develop, and are particularly distinct between those cells facing the zona pellucida. The blastocoele develops later, after further cleavage divisions have occurred. Small irregularly shaped cavities arise between two or three cells near the future abembryonic pole; at first, one or two cavities arise, but these eventually fuse to form the early blastocoele. The cells associated with the initial cavities develop pronounced junctional complexes between them. Continuous junctional complexes develop around the free borders of the trophoblast cells; in places the adjacent cell membranes are so close they appear to fuse, possibly giving rise to tight junctions.

The development of junctional complexes has also been described in the mouse.[6] So-called tight junctions were observed first in the morula stage.

Thus, there is good evidence that the appearance of the blastocoele is associated with the development of junctional complexes between the cells enveloping the blastocyst. In the words of Enders,[20]

> Formation of continuous junctional complexes around the free borders of the trophoblast cells can be considered the necessary prerequisite to blastocyst formation, since this process converts what is essentially an intercellular space into a space surrounded by an epithelium. It is at this point that the blastocyst becomes an organism with an external and internal environment rather than just a collection of cells.

When Does a Blastocoele Start to Form?

This question may at first seem unnecessary for under natural conditions the blastocyst develops at a certain time after fertilization. The question is much more meaningful, however, if restated in the form, "Does the blastocoele form only when the morula has reached some critical number of cells?" A cavity can be bounded by at least two flattened cells. The fewest number of cells known to be required to form a blastocyst under natural conditions is in fact two; this occasionally occurs in the elephant shrew *(Elephantulus myurus)*.[51] In many other species the blastocyst only forms in a morula consisting of many more cells. But comparative evidence of this kind does not demonstrate the importance of a critical number of cells, since a unique critical number could have been selected for each species during evolution. An unequivocal answer to the question can be obtained only if the cellular age of the morula can be varied experimentally within one species. In recent years the necessary experiments have been done in the mouse. Two techniques have been used. The first technique involves the reduction of the number of blastomeres in 2-, 4-, and 8-cell embryos.[44, 47] The results showed that blastulation begins at a fixed embryonic age, and not after a critical number of cells in the morula had developed. The second technique involves the fusion of early cleavage stages to form chimeras.[35, 45] Again, blastulation seems to occur at a fixed embryonic age since giant blastocysts were produced. With both techniques, no evidence of compensation to a critical cell number has been found. Thus, the development of the blastocoele depends on the interaction of an assembly of cells a fixed time after fertilization irrespective of the number of cells available. Recently Tarkowski, Witkowska and Nowiska[46] have produced parthenogenetic mouse blastocysts. Thus, the primary factors which regulate blastocyst formation are maternally derived.

How Does the Blastocoele Develop in an Eccentric Position?

It has already been pointed out that the asymmetry of the blastocyst arises from the segregation of two types of cells in the morula whose descendants form the inner cell mass and trophoblast respectively. Until recently, two theories concerning the differentiation of inner cell mass and trophoblast cells have been discussed: first, the theory that an organizing center exists in an undivided ovum which is essential for normal blastocyst development,[41] and second, the theory that cytoplasmic regions exist in the undivided ovum whose fate is determined.[38, 44] The latter theory involves bilateral symmetry and polarity in the egg.

The inadequacy of these theories has been shown by extensive experiments on the development of isolated blastomeres from 2-, 4-, and 8-cell mouse embryos.[47] Blastomeres were separated by treatment of the various stages with pronase; they were then cultured *in vitro* in a simple chemically defined medium.[5] The isolated blastomeres developed into trophoblastic vesicles, false blastocysts or blastocysts, the incidence varying with the type of blastomere cultured. Some of their results are summarized in Figure 1-5. Clearly the incidence of blastocysts diminishes with the stage of development and the number of blastomeres cultured, while the incidence of false blastocysts and trophoblastic vesicles increases. To explain these results Tarkowski and Wróblewska[47] postulate that the inner cell mass only differentiates if the morula

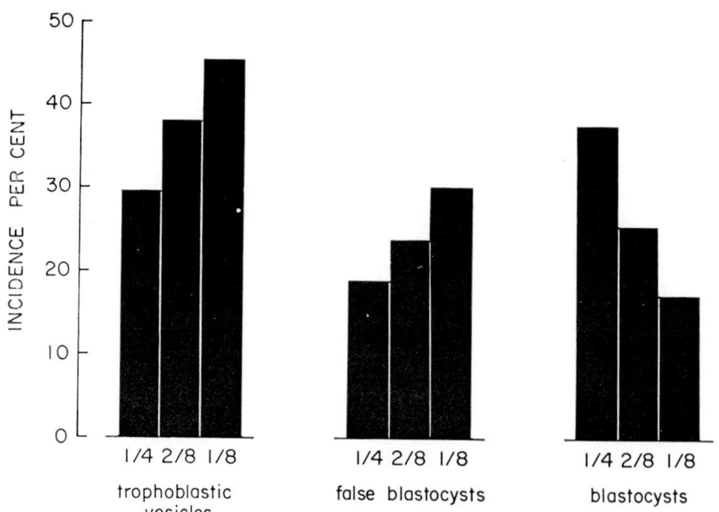

FIGURE 1-5. The incidence of trophoblastic vesicles, false blastocysts and normal blastocysts which develop *in vitro* from isolated and paired blastomeres (from Tarkowski and Wroblewska, 1967). ¼—beginning with one blastomere isolated from a 4-cell stage. 2⁄8—beginning with two blastomeres isolated from an 8-cell stage. ⅛—beginning with one blastomere isolated from an 8-cell stage.

contains sufficient number of cells to isolate some from the surrounding environment. In their own words:

> When a mouse egg passes from morula to blastocyst it is composed of about 30 cells. A certain number of these cells occupy the interior of the morula and are completely separated from outside by other cells. The latter become flattened and represent predecessors of the trophoblastic cells. It seems reasonable to assume that the conditions in which external and internal cells find themselves are diametrically different. The internal cells, being completely cut off from the interior, develop in a micro-environment created by external cells. In our opinion, the position of a cell in the morula and, a consequence of the position, the different environmental conditions play a decisive role in the differentiation of cells in one of the two directions (trophoblast versus inner cell mass). For the formation of the inner mass it is necessary that certain blastomeres should become isolated from the exterior before the moment when blastocoelic fluid starts to accumulate between the cells.

As far as we know no polarity exists in the mammalian embryo prior to the formation of the blastocyst, and the geometric location of the inner cell mass within the spherical blastocyst is randomly determined. The hypothesis of Tarkowski and Wróblewska[47] is attractive in that it attempts to explain the formation of the inner cell mass without invoking any prior spatial determinants in the embryo. However, it must not be forgotten that the blastocyst does acquire a polarity due to the development and location of the inner cell mass. Tarkowski and Wróblewska's hypothesis does not attempt to explain this polarity. Possibly a study of the interactions and the junctional complexes between the cells of the inner cell mass among themselves and with the trophoblast cells (Fig. 1-4c, II, III) may further our understanding of the organization and formation of the blastocyst.

FURTHER DEVELOPMENT OF THE BLASTOCYST

General Morphology

Soon after the blastocyst forms, a single layer of cells develops on the inner side of the inner cell mass. These cells are at least part of the presumptive endoderm cells and are called the *hypoblast*. The remainder of the inner cell mass, by analogy with the chick, is called the *epiblast.* The cells of the hypoblast proliferate and spread as a layer around the inside of the trophoblast; the sac that results within the blastocoele is called the *yolk sac.* Meanwhile the epiblast and hypoblast give rise to the *blastodisc* where the new embryo will develop. The layer of trophoblastic cells over the blastodisc is called *Rauber's layer.* The subsequent fate of Rauber's layer varies with the species. In some species the layer is lost, thus exposing the epiblast to the surface. This loss is known to occur in rabbits, ungulates, some insectivors and lemurs. In other species Rauber's layer persists. The behaviour of Rauber's layer has important consequences for the method of amnion formation.

Comparative Morphology of Amnion Formation in Mammals

In general, two mechanisms have evolved for formation of the amnion—fold formation and cavitation. Fold formation occurs when Rauber's layer is lost. Folds of the blastocyst wall arise around the edge of the blastodisc and envelop the early embryo. Fusion of the folds completes the formation of the amniotic sac in which the embryo lies. Da Costa[9] has named this mode of amnion formation *plectamnios.*

In species where Rauber's layer persists the amniotic cavity arises by the appearance of spaces between the cells of the inner cell mass. These spaces coalesce and eventually give rise to the amniotic sac by cavitation. Da Costa[9] named this method of amnion formation *schizamnios.* Many variations occur between species. For example, in some the cavity appears between the inner cell mass and the trophoblast, while in others the cavity arises entirely within the epiblast. Many examples of differences of species together with their evolutionary significance are discussed by Mossman.[36] In the remainder of this chapter we will give attention to amnion formation by cavitation since this appears to be the mechanism which occurs in man.

Amnion Formation in Man

At present we have only limited information on the formation of the amnion in man because of the few human embryos which

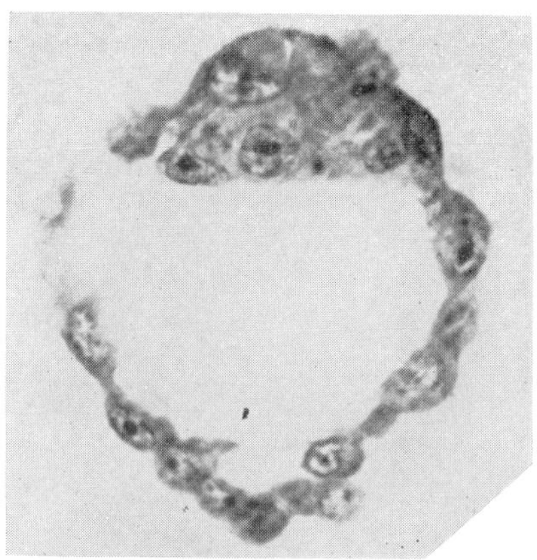

FIGURE 1-6a. Human blastocyst about 5 days old (from Hertig and Rock; Adams and Mulligan, 1954). ×550.

have been collected. Figure 1-6a shows a human blastocyst about 5 days old collected by Hertig *et al.*[25] The trophoblast and inner cell mass are clearly seen, but there is no indication of a space in the inner cell mass representing the early amniotic cavity. Figure 1-6b shows a human blastocyst attached to the decidua basalis on the uterus.[24] It is about 7.5 days old and the first signs of the amniotic cavity are present in the inner cell mass. Figure 1-6c shows a human embryo about 9 days old implanted in the endometrium.[24] A distinct amniotic cavity is present. These three specimens demonstrate that the amniotic cavity forms in the human embryo by cavitation about 7 days after conception. Unfortunately, the specimens are inadequate to study the detailed cytological processes involved. To obtain further cytological details we will turn to the monkey.

Amnion Formation in the Macaque

The formation of the amnion in the macaque has been described in great detail by Heuser and Streeter.[26] The first signs of the amnion appear on the tenth day of pregnancy. During the next three days the amnion and its cavity are completely formed. After the thirteenth day the amnion merely grows in size. For

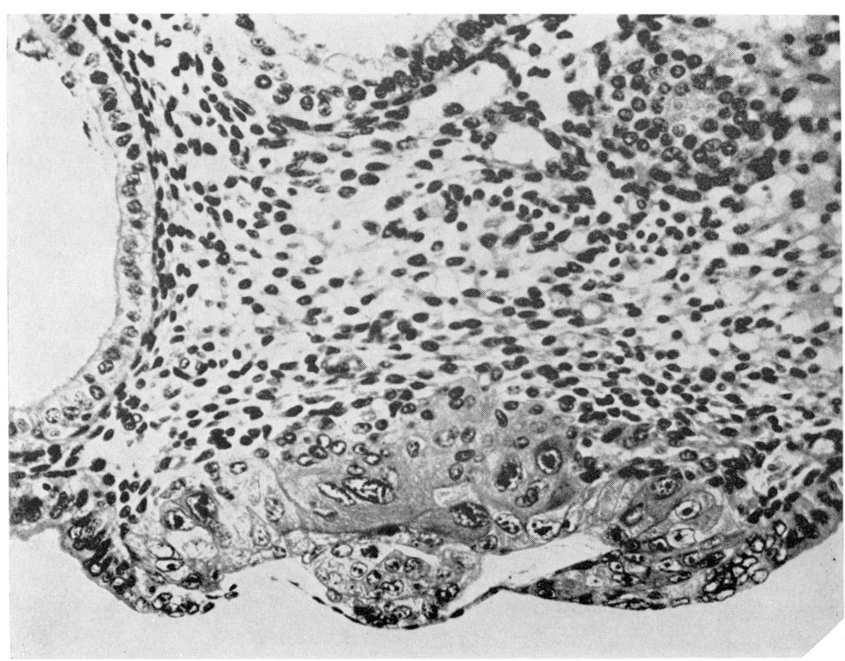

FIGURE 1-6b. Human blastocyst about 7½ days old attached to the decidua basalis (from Hertig and Rock, 1945). ×400.

convenience, Heuser and Streeter recognized four stages in the formation of the amnion (Figs. 1-7a, b, c, d).

The first stage is shown in Figure 1-7a from a 10-day-old embryo. The formative cells have given rise to a definite germ disc. Adjacent to the germ disc is a layer of amniogenic cells being delaminated from the trophoblast. The first sign of amniotic fluid appears in an intercellular space between the amniogenic cells and the germ disc. The second stage of amnion development is shown in Figure 1-7b from an 11-day-old embryo. The amniotic cells are clearly separated from the cytotrophoblast and have consolidated into a single-layered membrane of cuboidal cells. Laterally, the newly formed amnion is continuous with the germ disc. The amniotic cavity is well formed. The third stage of amnion development is shown in Figure 1-7c from an 11¾-day-old embryo. The amnion is distinctly separated from the trophoblast and a reticulum is developing between them. After the thirteenth

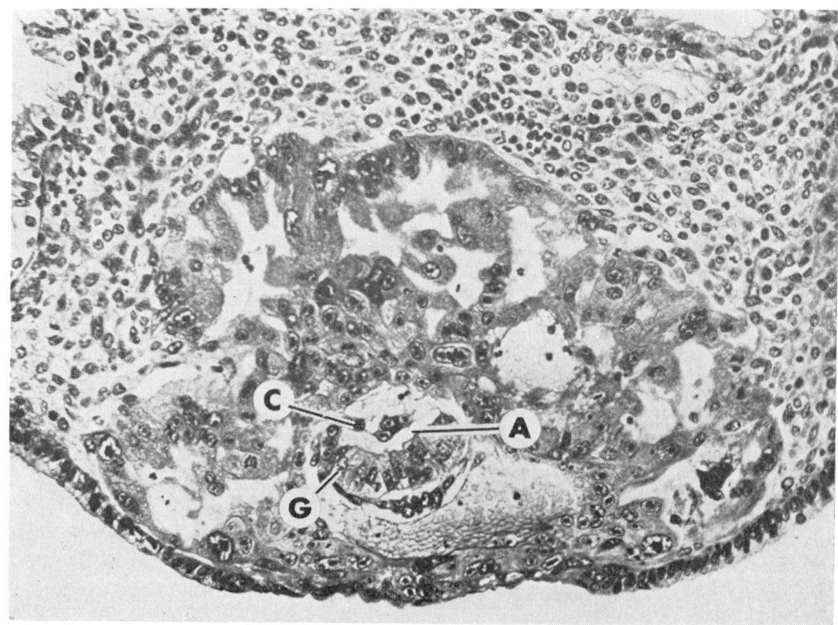

FIGURE 1-6c. Human embryo about 9 days old implanted in the endometrium (from Hertig and Rock, 1945). ×300. *A*, amniotic cavity. *C*, amniogenic cells. *G*, germ disc.

day the fourth stage is reached in which the amnion is fully formed (see Fig. 1-7d from a 17-day-old embryo).

Wall of the Early Amnionic Cavity and the Formation of Its Fluid

The studies on man and the macaque show that the wall of the amnion is derived from cells delaminated from the trophoblast. Unfortunately, very little is known about the ultrastructure of the amnion at early stages of development.[53] Furthermore, no study has been found on the ultrastructural features of amnion formation and the amniogenic cells.

In the early stages the amniotic cavity is bounded on one side by the cells delaminated from the trophoblast and on the other by the epiblast. Thus, the amniotic fluid could be derived initially from either the amnion or the germ disc. The latter possibility

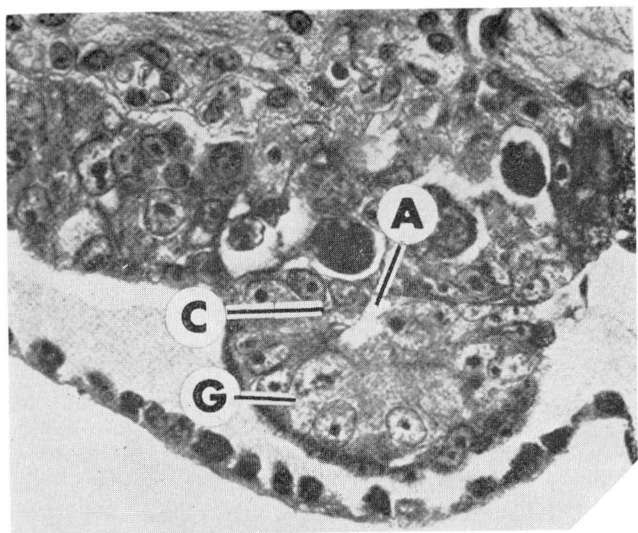

FIGURE 1-7a. Macaque blastocysts 10 days old (from Heuser and Streeter, 1941). ×500. *A*, amniotic cavity. *C*, amniogenic cells. *G*, germ disc.

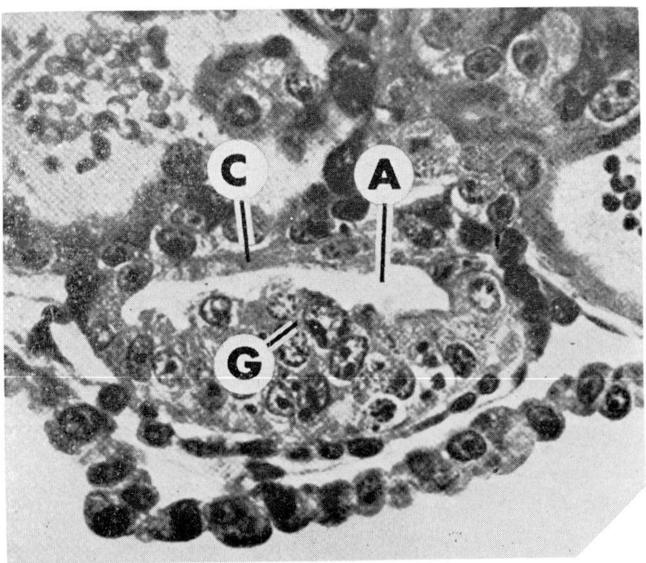

FIGURE 1-7b. Macaque blastocysts 11 days old (from Heuser and Streeter, 1941). ×500. *A*, amniotic cavity. *C*, amniogenic cells. *G*, germ disc.

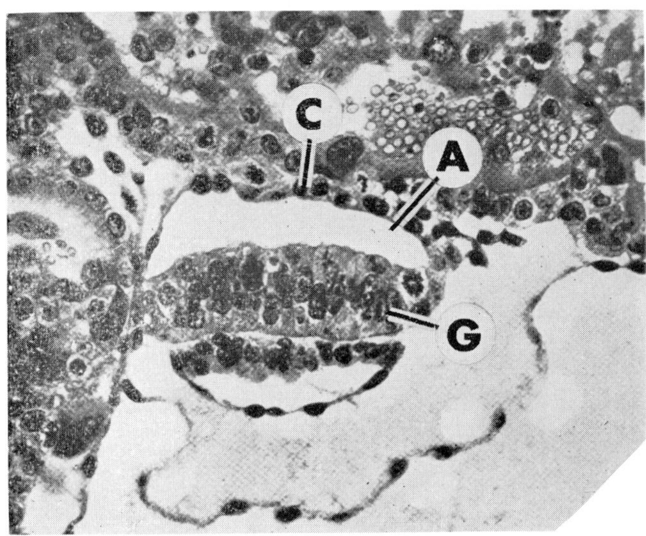

FIGURE 1-7c. Macaque blastocysts 11¾ days old (from Heuser and Streeter, 1941). ×300. *A*, amniotic cavity. *C*, amniogenic cells. *G*, germ disc.

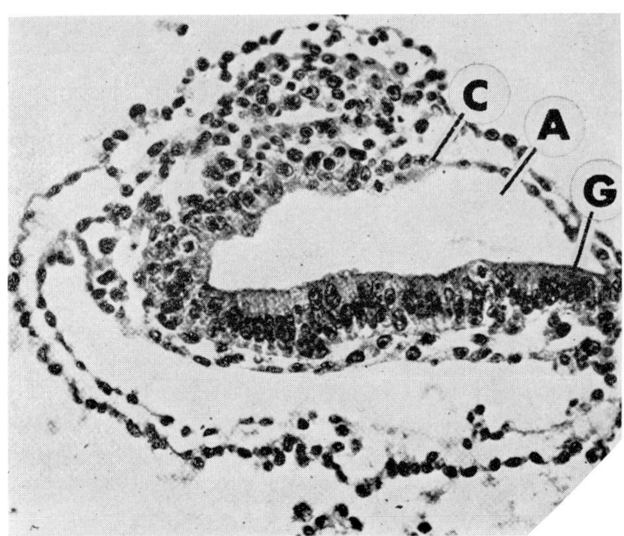

FIGURE 1-7d. Macaque blastocysts 17 days old (from Heuser and Streeter, 1941). × 200. *A*, amniotic cavity. *C*, amniogenic cells. *G*, germ disc.

was recognized by Heuser and Streeter.[26] It is important to realize that the formation of the amniotic fluid probably involves considerable fluxes of water and solutes from exogenous sources. If the fluid is transported through the early amnion it may be derived immediately from the maternal plasma via the trophoblast. If the fluid is transported through the germ disc it may be immediately derived from the blastocoele fluid. The latter phenomenon involves the passage of fluid between different compartments of the embryo and may be characterized by directional fluxes. We know nothing of these processes in early mammalian development. However, they are known to occur in early amphibian development, and have been studied in some detail by Tuft[48, 49] in *Xenopus laevis* with respect to the accumulation of fluid in the blastocoele and archenteron.

CONCLUSION

Our knowledge of amnion formation by cavitation is limited to classical morphological observations. In contrast, rapid progress is being made in the analysis of blastocyst formation, and it seems that similar approaches could be usefully applied to the study of amnion formation. The problems, however, could be more complex since by the time the amniotic cavity first appears the embryo has become compartmentalized, and it is necessary to consider the fluid fluxes between the various embryonic regions.

REFERENCES

1. Balinsky, B.I.: *An Introduction to Embryology,* 3rd ed. Philadelphia, Saunders, 1970.
2. Blandau, R.J.: *The Biology of the Blastocyst.* Chicago, University of Chicago, 1971.
3. Borghese, E., and Cassini, A.: Cleavage of mouse egg. In Rose, G.G. (Ed.): *Cinemicrography in Cell Biology.* New York, Academic Press, 1963.
4. Boyd, J.D., and Hamilton, W.J.: Cleavage, early development and implantation of the egg. In Parkes, A.S. (Ed.): *Marshall's Physiology of Reproduction,* 3rd ed. London, Longmans, 1952, Vol. II, pp. 1-126.
5. Brinster, R.L.: A method for *in vitro* cultivation of mouse ova from two-cell to blastocyst. *Exp Cell Res, 32:*205-208, 1963.

6. Calarco, P.G., and Brown, E.H.: An ultrastructural and cytological study of preimplantation development of the mouse. *J Exp Zool, 171:* 253-284, 1969.
7. Cole, R., and Paul, J.: Properties of cultural preimplantation mouse and rabbit embryos, and cell strains derived from them. In Wolstenholme, G.E.W. and O'Connor, M. (Eds.): *Preimplantation Stages of Pregnancy.* London, Churchill, 1965.
8. Corner, G.W.: The observed embryology of human single-ovum twins and other multiple births. *Am J Obstet Gynecol, 70:*933-951, 1955.
9. Da Costa, A.C.: Sur la formation de l'amnios chez les chéiroptères *(Miniopterus schreibersii)* et, en général, chez les mammifères. *Mem Soc portug Sci nat* (Seric biol No. 3), 1, 1920.
10. Cross, M.H.: Electrical properties of the short-circuited perfused rabbit blastocyst. *Proc Soc Study Reprod,* Boston, 1971.
11. Cross, M.H., and Brinster, R.L.: Transmembrane potential of the rabbit blastocyst trophoblast. *Exp Cell Res, 58:*125-127, 1969.
12. Cross, M.H., and Brinster, R.L.: Influence of ions, inhibitors and anoxia on transtrophoblast potential of rabbit blastocyst. *Exp Cell Res, 62:*303-309, 1970.
13. Curran, P.F.: Na, Cl, and water transport by rat ileum *in vitro. J Gen Physiol, 43:*1137-1148, 1960.
14. Dalq, A.M.: *Introduction to General Embryology.* New York, Oxford University, 1957.
15. Daniel, J.C.: Early growth of rabbit trophoblast. *Am Nat, 98:*85-98, 1964.
16. Diamond, J.M.: The mechanism of isotonic water transport. *J Gen Physiol, 48:*15-42, 1964.
17. Dick, D.A.T.: *Cell Water.* London, Butterworths, 1966.
18. Dickson, A.D.: The form of the mouse blastocyst. *J Anat, 100:*335-348, 1966.
19. Durbin, R.P.: Osmotic flow of water across permeable cellulose membranes. *J Gen Physiol, 44:*315-326, 1960.
20. Enders, A.C.: The fine structure of the blastocyst. In Blandau, R.J. (Ed.): *The Biology of the Blastocyst.* Chicago, University of Chicago, 1971, pp. 71-94.
21. Gamow, E., and Daniel, J.C.: Fluid transport in the rabbit blastocyst. *Wilhelm Rouse' Archiv, 164:*261-278, 1970.
22. No reference.
23. Hertig, A.T.: On the development of the amnion and exocoelomic membrane in the pre-villous human ovum. *Yale J Biol Med, 18:*107-115, 1945.
24. Hertig, A.T., and Rock, J.: Two human ova in the pre-villous stage, having a developmental age of about seven and nine days respectively. *Contr Embryol Carneg Inst, 31:*67-84, 1945.

25. Hertig, A.T., Rock, J., Adams, E.C., and Mulligan, W.J.: On the preimplantation stages of the human ovum: A description of four normal and four abnormal specimens ranging from the second to the fifth day of development. *Contr Embryol Carneg Inst, 35:*199-220, 1954.
26. Heuser, C.H., and Streeter, G.L.: Development of the macaque embryo. *Contr Embryol Carneg Inst, 29:*17-56, 1941.
27. Hubrecht, A.A.W.: Die Phylogenese des Amnions und die Bedeutung des Trophoblastes. *Verh Akad Wet Amst, 4:*1, 1895.
28. Kuhl, W.: Untersuchungen über die Cytodynamik der Furchung und Frühentwicklung des Eies der weisse Maus. *Abhandl Senckenb Naturforsch Ges, 456:*1-17, 1941.
29. Kuhl, W., and Friedrich-Freksa, H.: Richtungsköperbildung und Furchung des Eies sowie das Verhalten des Trophoblasten der weisse Maus. (Film). *Zool Anz (suppl) 9:*187-195, 1936.
30. Lewis, W., and Gregory, P.: Cinematographs of living developing rabbit eggs. *Science, 69:*226-229, 1929.
31. Lutwak-Mann, C.: Biochemical approach to the study of ovum implantation in the rabbit. *Mem Soc Endocrinol, No. 6:*35-49, 1959.
32. Lutwak-Mann, C.: Some properties of early embryonic fluids in the rabbit. *J Reprod Fertil, 1:*316-317, 1960.
33. Lutwak-Mann, C.: The rabbit blastocyst and its environment: Physiological and biochemical aspects. In Blandau, R.J. (Ed.): *The Biology of the Blastocyst.* Chicago, University of Chicago, 1971, pp. 243-260.
34. Lutwak-Mann, C., Boursnell, J.C., and Bennett, J.P.: Blastocyst-uterine relationships: Uptake of radioactive ions by the early rabbit embryo and its environment. *J Reprod Fertil, 1:*169-185, 1960.
35. Mintz, B.: Synthetic processes and early development in the mammalian egg. *J Exp Zool, 157:*85-100, 1964.
36. Mossman, H.W.: Comparative morphogenesis of the fetal membranes and accessory uterine structures. *Contrib Embryol Carneg Inst, 26:*129-246, 1937.
37. Mossman, H.W.: Orientation and site of attachment of the blastocyst: A comparative study. In Blandau, R.J. (Ed.): *The Biology of the Blastocyst.* Chicago, University of Chicago, 1971, pp. 49-57.
38. Mulnard, J.: Problèmes de structure et d'organisation morphogénétique de l'oeuf des Mammifères. In *Symposium on Germ Cells and Earliest Stages of Development.* Instituto Lombardo, Milan. Fondazione A. Baselli, 1961, pp. 639-688.
39. Mulnard, J.: Analyse microcinématographique du développement de l'oeuf de souris du stade II au blastocyste. *Arch Biol (Liege), 78:*107-138, 1967.
40. Schlafke, S., and Enders, A.C.: Cytological changes during cleavage and blastocyst formation in the rat. *J Anat, 102:*13-32, 1967.

41. Siedel, F.: Die Entwicklungsfähigkeiten isolierter Furchungszellen aus dem Ei des Kaninchens *Oryctolagus cuniculus. Roux Arch EntwMech, 152:*43-130, 1960.
42. Smith, M.S.: Active transport in the rabbit blastocyst. *Experientia, 26:* 736-737, 1970.
43. Spanner, D.C.: *Introduction to Thermodynamics.* New York, Academic Press, 1964.
44. Tarkowski, A.K.: Experimental studies on regulation in the development of isolated blastomeres of mouse eggs. *Acta Theriologica, 3:*191-267, 1959.
45. Tarkowski, A.K.: Mouse chimaeras developed from fused eggs. *Nature (Lond), 190:*857-860, 1961.
46. Tarkowski, A.K., Witkowska, A., and Nowicka, J.: Experimental parthenogenesis in the mouse. *Nature (Lond), 226:*162-164, 1970.
47. Tarkowski, A.K., and Wróblewska, J.: Development of blastomeres of mouse eggs isolated at the 4- and 8-cell stage. *J Embryol Exp Morphol, 18:*155-180, 1967.
48. Tuft, P.H.: Role of water-regulating mechanisms in amphibian morphogenesis: A quantitative hypothesis. *Nature (Lond), 192:*1049-1051, 1961.
49. Tuft, P.H.: The uptake and distribution of water in the embryo of *Xenopus laevis* (Daudin). *J Exp Biol, 39:*1-19, 1962.
50. Tuft, P.H., and Böving, B.C.: The forces involved in water uptake by the rabbit blastocyst. *J Exp Zool, 174:*165-172, 1970.
51. Van Der Horst, C.J.: Early stages in the embryonic development of Elephantulus. *S Afr J Med Sci, Biol (Suppl), 7:*55-65, 1942.
52. Waddington, C.H.: *New Patterns in Genetics and Development.* New York, Columbia University, 1962.
53. Wynn, R.M., and French, G.L.: Comparative ultrastructure of the mammalian amnion. *Obstet Gynecol, 31:*759-774, 1968.

Chapter 2

MECHANISMS OF INTRAUTERINE WATER TRANSFER IN PREGNANCY

A. Elmore Seeds

The tissue layers separating mother and fetus and enclosing amniotic fluid conform to the description of a partially semi-permeable membrane both *in vitro* and *in vivo.* These layers are readily permeable to water molecules and are also partially permeable to some but not all solutes.

The relative barrier to the diffusion of isotopic water presented by these tissue layers *in vitro* is given in Table 2-I.[11] Estimating

TABLE 2-I

	P_d *(cm sec^{-1})*
Amnion	2.88×10^{-4}
Chorion laeve	1.31×10^{-4}
Chorioamnion	1.31×10^{-4}

where P_d is the observed permeability of the isolated tissue layers.

the thickness of chorion laeve from the weight of a known area and assuming a specific gravity of 1.0, a diffusion coefficient (D) for THO (tritiated water) transfer across this tissue (0.6×10^{-5} cm^2/sec^{-1}) can be calculated and compared to the free diffusion coefficient of isotopic water at body temperature (3.0×10^{-5} cm^2/sec^{-1}). Such data indicate that isotopic water diffuses across this membrane approximately one fifth as rapidly as through an equivalent thickness of solvent water. Thus isotopic water crosses human placental tissue rapidly compared to equivalent layers of other biologic barriers, i.e. toad bladder,[8] $D = 5 \times 10^{-7}$ cm/ sec^{-1}, but placental tissue presents some resistance to THO diffusion when compared to an equivalent layer of water.

Based on both *in vitro* and *in vivo* observations, most solutes below a molecular weight of about 1000 are also able to cross these membranes, although not as rapidly as water, while larger molecules cannot cross this barrier except for a few specific situations probably involving a selective or active transport.[19]

DIFFUSION PERMEABILITY TO WATER

The permeability of placental tissue to isotopic water *in vitro* has been measured by calculating the transfer rate of THO across the membrane in response to a gradient in isotopic water and in the absence of any volume change in the two pools bathing the membrane, that is, any net transfer of water across the membrane (Fig. 2-1). Thus the labelled water is redistributed across the membrane only by random movements exchanging on a one-to-one basis with nonlabelled water molecules, and assuming that the isotopic water molecules behave as other unlabelled water molecules, this furnishes a measure of the membrane permeability

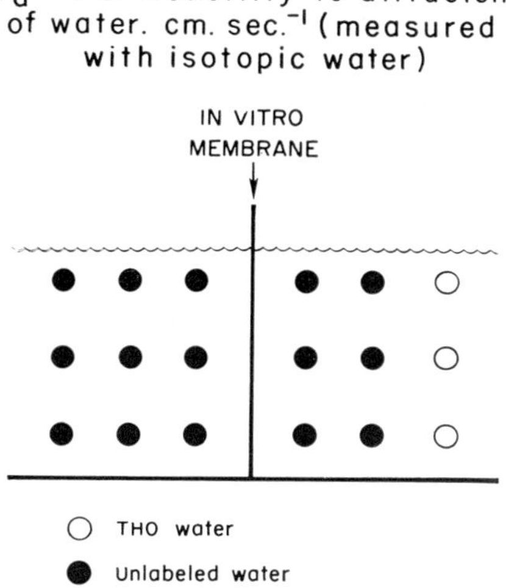

FIGURE 2-1. The diffusion permeability of human placental membranes to water (P_d) *in vitro* was measured as follows: An initial chemical potential gradient between two pools bathing the membrane was created by the addition of THO to chamber 1. The net transfer of THO from chamber 1 to chamber 2 in response to this isotopic water gradient and in the absence of any volume change in either chamber was used to calculate the diffusion permeability of these tissues to water (P_d).

to the diffusion of water. Such a permeability is indicated by P_d in units of cm/sec^{-1} and is measured using isotopic water.

OSMOTIC PERMEABILITY TO WATER

The net transfer of solvent water across placental membranes *in vitro* in response to a mole fraction difference in water concentration created by the addition of an osmotically active solute to one side of the system has been measured by means of volume changes in the two pools bathing the membrane.[18] The chemical potential difference or difference in water concentration across the membrane was approximated from the solute concentration difference (Fig. 2-2). Thus permeability to water transfer by osmosis was given in the same units of chemical potential as the diffusion permeability. However, the osmotic transfer rate exceeded the rate of isotope diffusion by 130 to 160 fold (Table

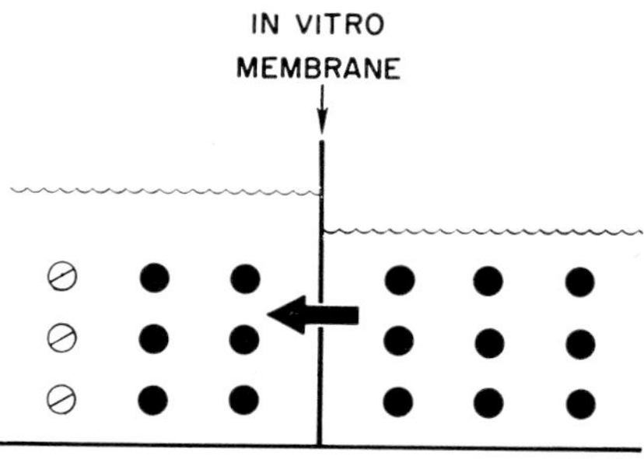

FIGURE 2-2. The osmotic permeability of human placental tissue to water (P_f) *in vitro* was measured as follows: An initial chemical potential gradient was created between the two pools bathing the membrane by the addition of Dextran-10 to chamber 2. These tissues are completely impermeable to Dextran-10. The rate of water transfer or osmosis from chamber 1 to chamber 2 in response to the osmotic gradient or difference in Dextran-10 concentration was measured by volume changes in the two pools and used to calculate the osmotic permeability (P_f) of this tissue to water.

2-II). Osmosis is thus a nondiffusional process across these tissues and the permeability to osmosis is frequently indicated by P_f or filtration permeability in cm/sec^{-1} (units identical to the diffusion permeabilities).

TABLE 2-II

Term amnion	P_d	=	2.88×10^{-4} cm/sec^{-1} (THO)
	P_f	=	3.73×10^{-2} cm/sec^{-1} (DEXTRAN-10)
Term chorion laeve	P_d	=	1.31×10^{-4} cm/sec^{-1} (THO)
	P_f	=	2.09×10^{-2} cm/sec^{-1} (DEXTRAN-10)

From Seeds, A. E.[18]

POROSITY OF PLACENTAL MEMBRANES

It has been previously shown by several investigators that water transfer across porous semipermeable artificial and biological membranes in response to osmotic or hydrostatic gradients proceeds at rates in excess of those predicted from the diffusion of isotopic water.[6, 9, 10, 12] This nondiffusional process is thought to result from the bulk movement of solvent through small porous channels and has been likened to the migration of water in a pipe in response to a pressure gradient, that is, a Poiseuille flow. The transfer of water across nonporous, artificial and biological membranes in response to osmotic or hydrostatic gradients proceeds at rates similar to those predicted from the diffusion of isotopic water.[15] Thus the observance of significant bulk flow across a membrane suggests the presence of pores or spaces within such tissue wherein the bulk structure of solvent water is unaltered.

The osmotic transfer of water across human amnion or chorion laeve *in vitro* at 130 to 160 fold the rate of diffusion of isotopic water across placental membranes indicates that, although the net transfer of water across multicellular tissue barriers such as the placenta takes place downhill in response to a chemical potential gradient, it is likely that the process is almost entirely nondiffusional, occurring principally by the bulk flow of solvent water through extracellular spaces or channels.

BULK FLOW OF WATER

Bulk flow, also termed laminar or Poiseuille flow, is the movement of solvent water in response to a difference in hydrostatic pressure similar to the movement of water through a pipe in response to a hydrostatic pressure gradient. Although such water movement in mass or in bulk form is directly proportional to the magnitude of the hydrostatic gradient, the rate of water transfer per unit gradient in chemical potential is many fold greater than the transfer rate of isotopic water in response to a difference in tracer water concentration.

Mauro[12] has shown that the nondiffusional flow of solvent water across a rigid, semipermeable collodion membrane in response to an osmotic gradient proceeds at a rate identical to that resulting from an equivalent hydrostatic pressure difference. This equivalent pressure is given by the osmolal difference in osmotically active solute on the two sides of the membrane, multiplied by the factor RT.

In other words, the osmotic force can be approximated assuming an impermeant solute from the van't Hoff equation:

$$\pi = mRT$$

where π = osmotic pressure (atmospheres)
m = molal concentration of solute (moles of solute/kg of water)
R = gas constant
T = absolute temperature (° Kelvin)

Thus a one milliosmolal solution of a nonpenetrating solute separated by a semipermeable barrier from pure solvent will result in the migration of water at the same rate as if a mechanical pressure of 25 cm of water has been applied to the pure solvent at room temperature. The permeability of such a membrane to the bulk transfer of solvent by osmotic or hydrostatic pressure can thus be described per unit of mechanical pressure or as a hydraulic conductivity. Hydraulic conductivities calculated from osmotic experiments for isolated human placental membranes at term are given in Table 2-III and compared to permeability of

TABLE 2-III

	Hydraulic Conductivity $\times 10^8$ *ml/sec/cm* H_2O/cm^2	Ratio: *Diffusion / Bulk Flow*
Amnion (Seeds[18])	2.58	1/130
Chorion laeve (Seeds[18])	1.46	1/160
Muscle capillary, hind limb of cat (Pappenheimer et al.[14])	2.5	
Toad bladder (Hays and Leaf[8])	.039	1/6
Toad bladder with vasopressin (Hays and Leaf[8])	1.52	1/115
Collodion III (Robbins and Mauro[16])	.72*	1/36
Collodion II (Robbins and Mauro[16])	5.4*	1/55
Collodion I (Robbins and Mauro[16])	160*	1/730

*units of ml/sec/cm H_2O

several biological and artificial membranes. It can be seen that as the permeability increases, the ratio of diffusional to nondiffusional flow increases. Theoretical considerations indicate that as pore size increases the diffusion of water increases by the square of the pore radius, while the bulk flow varies by the fourth power of the radius.

OSMOTIC EFFECTIVENESS OF PARTIALLY PERMEANT SOLUTES

A concentration difference in solute across a partially semipermeable membrane system can result in an osmotic transfer of water even when the barrier is readily permeable to this solute. If the readily penetrating solute does not cross this barrier as fast as water, it will exert some osmotic effect, albeit only a fraction of the ideal force observed with an impermeant solute.

Thus, although the human placenta is permeable to NaCl, glucose, and disaccharides, all of these compounds have been used experimentally *in vivo* to create concentration differences across the placenta, resulting in osmotic transfers of water between mother and fetus.

Studies in the human[2] demonstrated changes in the fetal extracellular solute and water content rapidly followed and paralleled maternal extracellular space alterations resulting from hypo or hypertonic infusions. The net transfer of water across the placenta between mother and fetus was suggested in these experiments by changes in fetal total osmotic pressure and sodium and total protein concentrations.

Bruns, Battaglia[3, 4] and co-workers first conclusively demonstrated transplacental water transfer in response to osmotic gradients in the rabbit and the primate rhesus monkey where a net decrease in fetal and/or amniotic fluid water resulted within one to two hours following hypertonic infusions containing NaCl or a disaccharide into the maternal circulation. Furthermore, a decrease in fetal water was measured following hypertonic disaccharide infusions into the amniotic cavity in these experiments. Other studies performed on pregnant rats have also demonstrated a net movement of water between mother and fetus in response to experimentally created osmotic gradients.[1, 20]

MECHANISM OF INTRAUTERINE WATER ACCUMULATION IN PREGNANCY

This type of experimental data suggests a possible mechanism for the physiologic net transfers of water occurring across the placental membranes and between intrauterine compartments in the intact animal during pregnancy. At term in the human, approximately 4 liters of water have accumulated within the uterus in the following spaces: fetus, 2800 ml, amniotic fluid, 800 ml, and placenta, 400 ml.

Since this quantity of water exceeds possible production from a fetal metabolic source, a large part of daily water requirements for normal fetal growth and development must be met by net transfers from the mother. Precisely how this water crosses the tissue layers separating mother and fetus to meet fetal requirements is still unknown, but a possible hypothesis is provided by the following lines of evidence: There are no experimental data *in vivo* or *in vitro* to indicate that water is actively transported across these membranes. Water crosses these tissue layers from an area of higher chemical potential to an area of lower chemical potential, and no net transfer occurs against a chemical potential gradient or in the absence of such a gradient.[3, 7, 11, 17] There is no evidence to date in the human to indicate the existence of a pumping mechanism that would result in the active transport of solute, such as sodium, across the placenta, followed by the passive migration of water.

However, water does cross these membranes in response to experimentally created osmotic gradients using many of the same solutes found in the biological fluids bathing these tissues *in vivo.* It has also been shown experimentally that water crosses these membranes in response to gradients in hydrostatic pressure.[5]

It can thus be suspected that the daily intrauterine water requirements in pregnancy may be satisfied by net transfers from the mother in response to hydrostatic or osmotic gradients. While looking for *in vivo* gradients to explain intrauterine water accumulation, it appears reasonable to consider gradients in chemical potential of water across only the placental cake, since most maternal/fetal exchange could be expected to occur at the site of maximum perfusion of intervening tissue layers provided by the apposition of maternal and fetal circulations. In addition, any net water transfer across the chorion laeve and amnion would be in a direction from amniotic fluid to maternal compartment, because of the decreased total solute and protein concentration present in amniotic fluid over the last half of pregnancy. Table 2-IV reviews measurements of *in vivo* gradients in hydrostatic and osmotic pressures across the placenta collected in experimental animals and in the human.

The total solute concentration of maternal and fetal blood are approximately equal. The colloid osmotic or oncotic pressure in fetal plasma is significantly below maternal values. Actual mechanical pressures due to the colloid concentration were measured in these experiments performed on maternal and fetal plasma collected in experimental animals and humans. A summary of hydro-

TABLE 2-IV

GRADIENTS IN OSMOTIC AND HYDROSTATIC PRESSURES ACROSS THE PLACENTA

Maternal	*Fetal*	*Species*
Total osmotic pressures (mOsm/kg H_2)		
289	289	Human
287	289	Human
303	300	Human
295.2 (uterine artery)	294.1 (umbilical artery)	Sheep and goats
297.2 (uterine vein)	294.3 (umbilical vein)	Sheep and goats
288 (intervillous space)	288 (umbilical vein)	Human
289.1 (arm vein)	292.7 (umbilical vein)	Human
Colloid osmotic pressures (mm H_2O)		
317	250	Goats
372	250	Sheep
356	305	Human*
Protein concentrations (gm %)		
6.5	4.5	Goat
7.8	4.5	Sheep
7.2	6.3	Human

Hydrostatic Pressures (mm Hg)

Intervillous Space	*Systolic Pressure, Umbilical Artery*	*Umbilical Vein*	*Species*
5			Rhesus monkey
	50	10	Sheep
	45-65	15-18	Sheep
	55-65	10.5	Sheep
12			Human
10			Human
6			Human
	75	26	Human
	80		Human
	48	24	Human
	88		Human

*From Hinckley, C. M., and Blechner, J. N.: Colloidal osmotic pressure of human maternal and fetal plasma. *Am J Obstet Gynecol, 103:*71, 1969. The remainder of the table from Seeds, A. E.: Water metabolism of the fetus. *Am J Obstet Gynecol, 92:*727, 1965.

static pressures measured *in vivo* on the two sides of the placenta are presented in Table 2-IV. Hydrostatic pressures on the two sides of the placenta in the human are difficult to measure accurately, however, from the very low pressures normally found in the intravillous space, and from measurements of transplacental hydrostatic gradients in animals the existence of a gradient that would transfer water from mother to fetus seems unlikely.

To summarize, (1) no gradient appears to exist in total solute concentration between mother and fetus; (2) any gradients in colloid osmotic pressure or in hydrostatic pressure appear to favor the transfer of water from fetus to mother, and thus do not help to explain intrauterine accumulation in pregnancy.

Despite the inability to demonstrate an osmotic or hydrostatic gradient between mother and fetus, it is still quite probable that intrauterine water requirements in pregnancy are supplied by such physicochemical forces, since experimentally water crosses these tissue layers in response to chemical potential gradients, and in the absence of such gradients no transfer takes place. Furthermore, because of the large placental surface area available for exchange and the relatively small daily requirements for intrauterine water accumulation, these needs can be easily met by gradients in chemical potential that are too small or too intermittent to be measured by present techniques.

MEMBRANE DISCRIMINATION BETWEEN SOLUTE AND SOLVENT

In trying to understand factors influencing the movement of water between maternal and intrauterine compartments across the placental membranes, and possibly to explain the apparent fetal water accumulation in the absence of a measurable chemical potential gradient *in vivo* favoring such an accumulation, a description of the partially semipermeable nature of the placental membranes is in order.

Placental membranes and other artificial and biological barriers have the ability to discriminate between permeating solute and solvent molecules. Thus, although urea crosses human chorion and amnion easily, this solute exerts a small osmotic force because it does not penetrate these membranes quite as rapidly as water. Other solutes penetrating these tissue layers also exert an osmotic force proportional to their relative permeating abilities. Thus, a solution containing a relatively impermeant solute molecule would exert an osmotic force close to the ideal mechanical pressure predicted by the van't Hoff equation. A solution containing a readily penetrating solute such as urea would exert only a small fraction of the ideal force. Another term may then be included in the van't Hoff relationship to describe the observed osmotic effect when using a permeating solute.

$\pi = \sigma$ nRT where $\sigma =$ reflection or Staverman coefficient.[21]

Sigma (σ) is, therefore, the ratio of the observed osmotic pressure to the ideal pressure predicted by the van't Hoff relationship if a nonpenetrating solute had been used. The reflection coefficient thus describes not only the osmotic effect of a solute, but also is a measure of the membranes' ability to discriminate between solvent molecules and the solute in question. Sigma is 1.0 for solutes not crossing a semipermeable membrane and approaches 0 for rapidly penetrating solutes.

This coefficient can also be included in permeability constants describing osmotic transfers. Thus, where P_d (2.88×10^{-4} cm/sec^{-1}) describes the diffusion of isotopic water across the amnion and P_f (3.73×10^{-2} cm/sec^{-1}) describes the migration of solvent water due to osmosis or to a concentration difference of an impermeant solute (Dextran-10) on the two sides of the membrane, σP_f would describe the osmotic water transfer resulting from a concentration difference of a solute able to penetrate the amnion. That is, σP_f would represent observed transfer rate where σ represents the ratio of the observed rate to the rate (P_f) expected had the membrane been completely impermeant to solute. Table 2-IV presents the observed permeability constants across amnion and chorion laeve measured for osmotic water transfer in response to a concentration difference of several small, partially penetrating solutes. Sigma for these solutes can be calculated by dividing the observed value by the ideal transfer rate measured with an impermeant solute. Reflection coefficients calculated in this fashion for these solutes across the *in vitro* human amnion and chorion laeve are summarized in Table 2-V.

TABLE 2-V

OSMOTIC EFFECTIVENESS OF PARTIALLY PENETRATING SOLUTES

	Amnion		*Chorion*	
Solute	P_f ($\times 10^2$ cm/sec $^{-1}$)	σ	P_f ($\times 10^2$ cm/sec $^{-1}$)	σ
Urea	.064 (5)	.02	.014 (3)	.01
NaCl	.136 (3)	.04	.032 (3)	.02
Glucose	.218 (5)	.06	.11 (3)	.05
Sucrose	.243 (4)	.07	.11 (5)	.05
Dextran	3.73 (25)		2.09 (16)	

From Seeds, A. E.[18]

The reflection coefficients of these solutes are of considerable biological significance. The macromolecules such as the serum proteins, since they cannot cross many body membranes, have a reflection coefficient of 1.0, and thus exert an osmotic pressure of 26.2 cm H_2O/mOsm at body temperature across impermeable membranes. Urea, with a reflection coefficient of 0.02, would exert an osmotic pressure of only about 0.5 cm H_2O/mOsm across the amnion, or one-fiftieth of the ideal effect. This accounts for the importance of the serum colloid osmotic pressure or that portion of the osmotic force due to the serum macromolecules, i.e. proteins. As shown by Meschia and Setnikar,[13] water can be transferred by osmosis across a partially semipermeable membrane against an apparent vapor pressure or activity gradient predicted by the colligative properties of the two solutions bathing the membrane. This passive transfer of water from a solution of higher concentration to a less concentrated solution occurs if the solute present in higher concentration crosses the membrane more easily than the solute present in lower concentration. Thus, to calculate the correct gradient in osmotically active solute existing across such a membrane and to predict the direction and rate of water transfer, not only the solute concentrations but also the reflection coefficients describing the relative penetrating abilities of these solutes must be known. Although no difference in total solute concentration appears to exist across the placenta, it is apparent that an osmotic gradient may still be present if different proportions of specific solutes with separate reflection coefficients are present on the two sides.

Significant bulk flows across partially semipermeable membranes such as placental tissue are accompanied by solvent drag. When water crosses this tissue by bulk flow, the transfer of solute molecules contained in the moving stream will be accelerated in the direction of the flow and retarded in the opposite direction. This is known as the solvent drag effect and is most pronounced for solutes crossing these membranes principally by the same extracellular pathway as water.

In Vivo Significance of Porous, Partially Semipermeable Nature of Placental Membranes

Further clarification of the *in vivo* significance of bulk flow and other closely related phenomena, such as solvent drag and membrane discrimination between solute and solvent, is gained from separating intrauterine water circulation in pregnancy into the two following categories:

1. The gradual accumulation of 4 liters of water within the uterus over a nine-month period represents the long-term, net uptake picture. The maximum rate of increase in water sometime near term is only approximately 30 cc/day. The role of bulk flow in the transfer of such small quantities of water may be small.

2. However, there is indirect evidence that significant bulk flows are taking place between maternal, fetal, and amniotic fluid compartments, even though the total solute and water contents of these compartments are changing very slowly with time in the steady state situation. This topic is discussed in the following chapter, but briefly, the low protein and total solute concentration of term amniotic fluid results in a significant osmotic gradient

between either the fetal or maternal compartment and the amniotic cavity across such possible exchange surfaces as amnion, chorion laeve, and/or fetal skin. In addition, the fetus has been reported to swallow approximately 450 cc of amniotic fluid per hour, which is presumably reabsorbed from the GI tract, and to excrete a very hypotonic urine in amounts probably in excess of 450 cc/day. Since the amniotic fluid total solute concentration is only slightly hypotonic ($\cong$ 255-270 mOsm/liter) at term, a significant quantity of free water must be reabsorbed from this space via some other pathway of exchange with fetal or maternal compartments.

In summary, water requirements for normal intrauterine growth and development of the fetus are most likely satisfied by net transfers aross the placenta from the mother in response to osmotic or hydrostatic gradients that are too small or too intermittent to measure. Much larger net transfers of water between amniotic fluid and adjacent fetal and maternal compartments are probably occurring during near steady state conditions at term in response to similar gradients. Water transfer across the *in vitro* placental membranes in response to osmotic or hydrostatic gradients occurs at rates many times in excess of those predicted from the diffusion of isotopic water, suggesting that *in vivo* water transfer may occur by nondiffusional bulk flow in response to similar gradients. The osmotic effect of different solutes varies inversely with their ability to cross the placental membranes, and although the most active osmotic solutes are the impermeant macromolecules, even such a small and readily permeating solute as urea exerts some osmotic force, since it does not penetrate these membranes as rapidly as water.

REFERENCES

1. Adolph, E.F., and Hoy, P.A.: Regulation of electrolyte composition of fetal rat plasma. *Am J Physiol, 204:*392, 1963.
2. Battaglia, F.C., Prystowsky, H., Smisson, C., Hellegers, A.E., and Bruns, P.D.: Effect of the administration of fluids intravenously to mothers upon the concentrations of water and electrolytes in plasma of human fetuses. *Pediatrics, 25:*2, 1960.

3. Bruns, P.D., Hellegers, A.E., Seeds, A.E., Behrman, R.E., and Battaglia, F.C.: Effects of osmotic gradients across the primate placenta upon fetal and placental water contents. *Pediatrics, 34:*407, 1964.
4. Bruns, P.D., Linder, R.O., Drose, V.E., and Battaglia, F.C.: The placental transfer of water from fetus to mother following the intravenous infusion of hypertonic mannitol to the maternal rabbit. *Am J Obstet Gynecol, 86:*160, 1963.
5. Dancis, J., Brenner, M.A., and Money, W.L.: Some factors affecting the permeability of the guinea pig placenta. *Am J Obstet Gynecol, 84:*570, 1962.
6. Durbin, R.P., Frank, H., and Solomon, A.K.: Water flow through frog gastric mucosa. *J Gen Physiol, 39:*535, 1956.
7. Garby, L.: Studies on transfer of matter across membranes with special reference to the isolated human amniotic membrane and the exchange of amniotic fluid. *Acta Physiol Scand, 40:* (Suppl, 137), 1957.
8. Hays, R.M., and Leaf, A.: Studies on the movement of water through the isolated toad bladder and its modification by vasopressin. *J Gen Physiol, 45:*905, 1962.
9. Hevesy, G., Hofer, E., and Krogh, A.: The permeability of the skin of frogs to water as determined by D_2O and H_2O. *Skand Arch Physiol, 72:* 199, 1935.
10. Koefoed-Johnson, V., and Ussing, H.H.: The contributions of diffusion and flow to the passage of D_2O through living membranes. *Acta Physiol Scand, 28:*60, 1953.
11. Lloyd, S.J., Garlid, K.D., Reba, R.C., and Seeds, A.E.: Permeability of different layers of the human placenta to isotopic water. *J Appl Physiol, 26:*274, 1969.
12. Mauro, A.: Nature of solvent transfer in osmosis. *Science, 126:*252, 1957.
13. Meschia, G., and Setnikar, I.: Experimental study of osmosis through a colloidion membrane. *J Gen Physiol, 42:*429, 1958.
14. Pappenheimer, J.R., Renkin, E.M., and Borrero, L.M.: Filtration, diffusion, and molecular sieving through peripheral capillary membranes. A contribution to the pore theory of capillary permeability. *Am J Physiol, 167:*13, 1951.
15. Price, H.D.: The Water Permeability of Lipid Bilayer Membranes. Ph.D. Dissertation. Baltimore, Johns Hopkins University, 1969, pp. 131-32.
16. Robbins, E., and Mauro, A.: Experimental study of the independence of diffusion and hydrodynamic permeability coefficients in collodion membranes. *J Gen Physiol, 43:*523, 1960.
17. Scoggin, W.A., Harbert, G.M., Anslow, W.P., Van't Riet, B., and McCaughey, H.S. Jr.: Feto-maternal exchange of water at term. *Am J Obstet Gynecol, 90:*7, 1964.
18. Seeds, A.E.: Osmosis across term human placental membranes. *Am J Physiol, 219:*551, 1970.

19. Seeds, A.E.: Placental transfer. In Barnes, A.C. (Ed.): *Intrauterine Development*. Philadelphia, Lea and Febiger, 1968, p. 103.
20. Seller, M.J.: The effect of maternal overhydration on the rat fœtus. *J Exp Physiol, 48*:292, 1963.
21. Staverman, A.J.: The theory of measurement of osmotic pressure. *Rec Trav Chim des Pays-Bas, 70*:344, 1951.

Chapter 3

AMNIOTIC FLUID

A. Elmore Seeds

Formation of the amniotic sac occurs early in pregnancy, and by the ninth week it is the major fluid space surrounding the developing fetus. The chorionic cavity and yolk sac have almost disappeared at this stage, and a significant allantoic sac never develops during human placentation.

AMNIOTIC FLUID VOLUME, MEASUREMENTS AND SIGNIFICANCE

Measurements of amniotic fluid accumulation throughout pregnancy are summarized in Table 3-I. Volumes of 5 to 10 cc have

TABLE 3-I

AMNIOTIC FLUID VOLUME

Period of Gestation (wk)	*Mean Volume ml*	*Range*	*No. of Observations*
8-15	103	(3.2-360)	7
	89	(5-245)	30
	83	(10.5-180)	11
	59	(10-135)	17
15-25	167	(115-362)	7
	270	(70-573)	11
	238	(54-500)	11
	251	(149-365)	6*
37	687	(229-1,338)	7
38	1,032	(533-1,512)	9
39	841	(221-1,296)	10
40	791	(330-1,455)	8
41	636	(172-1,231)	10
42	324	(0-441)	10
43	244	(77-438)	5

*From Gadd, R. L.[14] Remainder of table from Seeds, A. E.[38]

been reported as early as eight weeks[48, 50] and the amount increases rapidly thereafter proportional to fetal growth and gestational age until close to term.[13, 14, 16, 30] Differences between investigators are apparent in Table 3-I, but each series shows a serial increase in amniotic fluid volume with gestational age. Some of the data suggest that this increase is an exponential function of gestational age, fetal heel-toe, or crown-rump length; however, a recent study contends that fluid volume increases linearly with increases in heel-toe length of the fetus or gestational age.[12]

Serial measurements[13, 14, 15] indicate that a maximum volume of amniotic fluid of approximately 1000 cc is obtained just prior to term at 38 to 39 weeks' gestational age, and subsequently a serial diminution in the amount of fluid takes place (Fig. 3-1), so that after 42 weeks the mean volumes fall below 300 ml. It has been postulated that this decrease in fluid volume corresponds to diminution in placental function. The postmature syndrome, i.e. babies born significantly beyond their expected date of confinement with evidence of chronic hypoxia, meconium staining and/or stillborn, is accompanied by a lack of amniotic fluid or oligohydramnios.[27] Evidence has also been reported that patients with

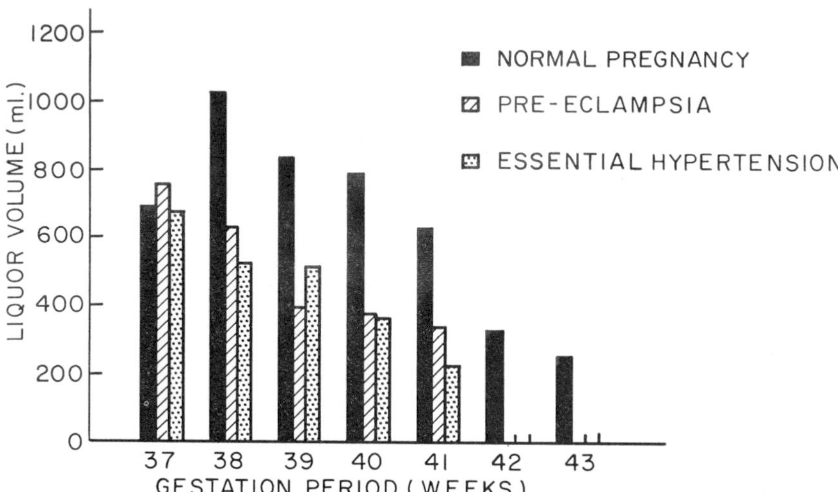

FIGURE 3-1. Mean amniotic fluid volumes at various periods of gestation. (From Elliott and Inman.[13])

preeclampsia and essential hypertension experience an earlier onset of the postmature syndrome and concomitant reduction in amniotic fluid. However, evaluation of such fluid volume changes becomes much more complex when the following facts are considered: During the period of 38 to 42 weeks' gestational age, amniotic fluid is decreasing, accompanied by no evidence of an increase in fetal hypoxia or distress *in utero.* There is no significant increase in perinatal morbidity and mortality until after 42 weeks.[27] Several clinical conditions associated with a high incidence of fetal hypoxia and suspected placental malfunction (i.e. diabetes, erythroblastosis, preeclampsia) also have an increased incidence of hydramnios[13, 14, 31, 53] (Table 3-II), although one

TABLE 3-II

ASSOCIATED COMPLICATIONS OF PREGNANCY IN SEVENTY-FOUR PATIENTS WITH HYDRAMNIOS*

Complications	*Patients*		*Total Incidence At Hospital*
	No.	*%*	*%*
Diabetes mellitis	14	18.9	0.42
Preeclampsia	11	14.9	4.5
Hypertensive vascular disease	2	2.7	1.6
Heart disease	2	2.7	1.5
Rh incompatibility	5	6.8	..
Psychiatric disease	4	5.4	..
Fibromyomas of uterus	2	2.7	..
Epilepsy	2	2.7	..
Anemia	2	2.7	..
Thyrotoxicosis	1	1.4	..
Late latent lues	1	1.4	..
Hypothyroidism	1	1.4	..
Intercapillary glomerulosclerosis	1	1.4	..
Kyphoscoliosis with atelectasis	1	1.4	..
Pyelonephritis	1	1.4	..
Hyperemesis gravidarum	1	1.4	..
Mucous colitis	1	1.4	..
Adrenal cortical hypofunction	1	1.4	..
Total	53	..	..

*In 43 of these patients, history, laboratory findings, and results were normal.

Table from Moya, F., and co-workers.[31]

recent study[14] did contend that no significant increase in amniotic fluid volume accompanied moderate preeclampsia and a marked reduction in volume occurred with severe preeclampsia.

The physiological significance of amniotic fluid volume increases remains obscure. It can be postulated that the steady expansion of this fluid compartment with gestational age provides a stimulus to uterine growth and enlargement and perhaps provides a partially weightless environment for the fetus.[51] Volume changes near term have also been cited as possible factors leading to cervical ripening and/or the initiation of labor, although recent data suggest that the volume is diminishing at the time when normal labor usually commences.

ORIGIN OF AMNIOTIC FLUID

The parallel increase in fetal size and amniotic fluid volume suggests that this pool may in part originate from the fetus. Changes in amniotic fluid composition over the last half of pregnancy indicate that fetal urine may provide a major source for fluid production during this period.[38] In addition, it has recently been shown that prior to keratinization, at about 24 to 26 weeks' gestational age, fetal skin is very permeable to the diffusion of isotopic water.[32] Early in pregnancy permeability values for fetal skin *in utero* are similar to those measured across isolated amnion and chorion laeve, suggesting that this well-vascularized surface area separating fetal from amniotic fluid compartments may function as a significant exchange site at this stage in gestation. Thus, even early in pregnancy a significant proportion of this fluid may be a product of the fetal compartment.

AMNIOTIC FLUID COMPOSITION

Studies of amniotic fluid composition early in pregnancy (Tables 3-III and 3-IV have led to the conclusion that this pool is a dialysate of maternal and/or fetal fluids.[38] The concentrations of total solute and small diffusable crystalloid molecules were very similar to those found in maternal and fetal plasma, with the exception of an increased chloride concentration.[44] Amniotic fluid protein

TABLE 3-III

COMPOSITION OF AMNIOTIC FLUID AND MATERNAL AND FETAL BLOOD

Amniotic Fluid	*No. of Cases*	*T. O. P. (mOsm/liter)*	*Na (mEq/liter)*	*Cl (mEq/liter)*	*K (mEq/liter)*	*NPN (mg %)*	*Urea (mg %)*	*Uric acid (mg %)*	*Creatinine (mg %)*	*Total Protein (gm %)*	*Total Lipid (mg %)*	*Water Content (%)*
2-4 Months	8	291	131	110		27			1.43	0.24		98.7
	4	286.7	137.4		4.0							
	38			106		20.3	20.6			0.20		
	6	280					34					
							20.7	2.8	1.04			
4-6 Months	23			106		25.4	26.0			0.25		
	8	277					37					
		280										
							19.4	3.6	1.06			
2-6 Months*			135	118	4.3		19		1.4	0.436		
6-8 Months	10			106		26.5	27.4			0.26		
	5	260					40					
		273										
							31.1	5.6	2.2			
9 Months	7	259.4		106		23			2.30	0.22		
(term)	8	256										
	21	270.2	127	106		27				0.23		98.8
		256										
	9	265.5	125.3		4.0							
	65			106		31.8	33.9			0.31		
			127	103	4.0		29		2	0.26	48	
	14	251					44					
	17	271										

TABLE 3-III

COMPOSITION OF AMNIOTIC FLUID AND MATERNAL AND FETAL BLOOD

Amniotic Fluid	*No. of Cases*	*T. O. P. (mOsm/liter)*	*Na (mEq/liter)*	*Cl (mEq/liter)*	*K (mEq/liter)*	*NPN (mg %)*	*Urea (mg %)*	*Uric acid (mg %)*	*Creatinine (mg %)*	*Total Protein (mg %)*	*Total Lipid (gm %)*	*Water Content (%)*
							36.1	6.8	3.7			
Hydramnios			131	110	5.0					0.64		
	4		138		3.7							
Maternal	7	289		106		22				6.8		
serum, term	9	281										
pregnancy	21	296	136	103		24			1.55	6.1		91.6
	9	289.1	138		3.5							
	65			106		20.3	20.7			6.6		
	25										1,018	
	35	288										
							24.9	3.57	1.02			
Fetal serum,	13	289.1										
term	7	289		106		19				5.2		
pregnancy	10	292.7	140		4.5							
	65			106		26.2	25.9			5.7		
	29										198	
	35	288										

*From Sinha, R., and Carlton, M.[44] Remainder of table from Seeds, A. E.[38]

concentration, between 200 and 300 mg % was significantly below maternal and fetal plasma levels at this stage in pregnancy. The ph, P_{CO_2} and bicarbonate concentration of this fluid are closest to maternal and fetal plasma levels early in pregnancy.[41]

These findings indicate that amniotic fluid early in pregnancy is very similar in composition to other body extracellular fluids (interstitial, cerebrospinal) considered to be dialysates of plasma across membranes readily permeable to the small molecular weight solutes and impermeable to the larger molecular weight proteins and lipids. Thus, most solutes including electrolytes diffuse into these pools to achieve concentrations equivalent to those found in plasma. However, since only a small amount of anionic protein gets into such fluid, an excess of chloride anion passively diffuses into these compartments to preserve electrochemical neutrality, resulting in an increased chloride concentration, i.e. Gibbs-Donnen equilibrium. Thus, early in pregnancy the low protein and lipid content, correspondingly high chloride and water concentration, and concentrations of other solutes and pH similar to maternal and fetal plasma strongly suggest that this fluid originates as a dialysate of maternal and/or fetal fluids. The increase in amniotic fluid carbon dioxide tension in late pregnancy is most likely secondary to elevations in fetal and maternal uterine vein P_{CO_2}s with advancing gestational age. The decrease in amniotic fluid bicarbonate concentration is in part secondary to the excretion of fixed acids by the fetal kidney near term and also secondary to the increasing hypotonicity of this fluid compartment over the last half of gestation. A fetal urine pH of 6.2 has been reported near term.[26]

The following evidence has been used to infer a significant contribution by the fetal kidney to amniotic fluid formation over the last half of pregnancy:

1. A progessive decrease in amniotic fluid total solute concentration takes place from the twentieth week until term in humans (Table 3-III) (Fig. 3-5) and in the rhesus monkey.[4, 8, 24, 39]

2. Studies of fetal urine production *in utero* have shown a progressive decrease in tonicity with increasing gestational age.[3] In addition, fetal urine collected *in utero* near term in experi-

TABLE 3-IV

pH, P_{CO_2}, AND BICARBONATE CONCENTRATION IN HUMAN AMNIOTIC FLUID THROUGHOUT PREGNANCY

*Gestational Age**		*H+(mEq/liter)*	*pH*	P_{CO_2} *(mm Hg)*	HCO_3 *(mM/liter)*
10-23 weeks	mean	59.34	7.227	41.1	16.57
(28)	± S.E.M.	±1.25		±0.5	±0.37
25-31 weeks	mean	67.81	7.169	43.2	15.16
(8)	± S.E.M.	±2.99		±1.4	±0.63
Term	mean	78.45	7.105	50.8	14.82
(12)	± S.E.M.	±2.68		±0.9	±0.56

*Number of observations in parentheses.

Table from Seeds, A. E., and Hellegers, A. E.[41]

TABLE 3-V

AVERAGE VALUES OBTAINED IN BLADDER SAMPLES IN THREE FOETAL AGE-RANGES IN THE SHEEP*

Foetal Age (days)	*Osmotic Pressure (mOsm/liter)*	*Total N (mg/100 ml)*	*Urea (mg/100 ml)*	*Creatinine (mg/100 ml)*	*Total Phosphorous (mg/100 ml)*	Na^+ *(mEq/liter)*	Cl^- *(mEq/liter)*	K^+ *(mEq/liter)*
81- 93	239	76	102	3	9	81	67	4
104-117	207	110	123	6	2	71	47	4
130-142	116	180	287	27	3	26	21	8

*From Alexander, D. P., and Nixon, D. A.[2]

mental animals (Table 3-V) or urine excreted within a few minutes of delivery in the human, and presumably formed *in utero,* is markedly hypotonic (T. O. P. $\cong$ 80-140 mOsm/liter) to either maternal or fetal plasma.[2, 24, 25]

3. The concentrations of urea, uric acid, and creatinine, excreted in fetal urine in considerably higher concentrations near term than that of fetal or maternal blood,[2, 3, 25] are significantly increased during the last trimester in amniotic fluid (Table 3-IV).[47]

4. Placental membranes are readily permeable to those small molecular weight solutes.[28, 29]

5. Amniotic fluid taurine concentrations have been shown to rise steadily in rhesus monkey amniotic fluid while the concentrations of other amino acids are decreasing.[22] Taurine has also been shown to be elevated in newborn urine.[52]

6. There is a high correlation between renal agenesis and oligohydramnios in the last part of pregnancy.[21]

7. Amniotic fluid becomes steadily more acidic with increasing gestational age (Table 3-IV), and a low pH has been measured in fetal urine near term.[26]

Thus, the large amniotic fluid volumes later in pregnancy would appear to be principally the result of fetal urine excretion.

FETAL URINE PRODUCTION

Fetal urine production and composition have been studied in experimental animals and in humans with somewhat conflicting results. Analyses of urine collected in the human fetus at birth and from the exteriorized sheep fetus with intact placental circulation showed the formation of a markedly hypotonic fluid near term. The total solute concentration was 80-140 mOsm/liter and production rates in the sheep at term were 0.04 ml/min/kg.[2, 3, 24, 25] Recently, however, studies in fetal rhesus monkeys *in utero* and in exteriorized fetal sheep have shown the production of a more concentrated urine.[10, 45] Production rates of 0.05-0.08 ml/min/kg of urine, with a mean total solute concentration in the more recent studies of 271 mOsm/kg, suggested the addition of approximately 200-400 ml urine/day in the human very similar in tonicity to that found in normal amniotic fluid near term.

Evaluation of these contrasting descriptions of fetal urine production remains difficult since all of the studies were carefully performed by reliable workers, with evidence in most instances of nonstressed experimental preparations. Nevertheless, a possible explanation for the discrepancies may be derived from the following observations:

1. In experimental preparations wherein the bladder was surgically exposed and catheterized in the exteriorized sheep fetus for serial collection of fetal urine samples, only the initial urine samples were consistently hypotonic in near-term fetuses.[3] Urine subsequently collected in these experiments became hypertonic and remained in this range throughout the experiment. It would appear that the stress of the experimental procedure led to the production of a more concentrated urine. An inverse relationship was observed between urine volume and solute concentration in that the urine volume produced was lowest during periods of high total solute concentration.

2. Measurements of fetal urine volume near term in these experiments were always performed during periods when relatively concentrated urine was collected even in the studies where the initial bladder sample was hypotonic.[3, 10, 45]

3. Urine in the human newborn collected immediately at birth and presumably formed *in utero* is markedly hypotonic to maternal and fetal plasma, but shortly after birth this urine becomes slightly hypertonic.[25] Such findings indicate that there is an increase in fetal urine total solute concentration in response to the stress of delivery.

Therefore, fetal urine formed *in utero* near term in the nonstressed fetus is most likely markedly hypotonic and produced in large volumes, probably in excess of the amniotic fluid swallowed by the fetus. This dilute urine is accurately measured by immediate collection of bladder samples in the newborn, but any exposure to stress, such as exteriorization of the fetus or the surgical procedures attendant to bladder and ureteral catheterization, results in an immediate increase in total solute concentration and reduction in urine volume probably secondary to the release of antidiuretic hormone. Accurate measurement of fetal urine volume production near term would appear to be very difficult in view of the ease with which urine concentrating mechanisms are activated by experimental manipulation.

SITES OF SOLUTE AND WATER EXCHANGE BETWEEN AMNIOTIC FLUID AND FETUS

The relatively narrow range in total solute concentration of this fluid (255-270 mM/liter) at term, slightly hypotonic compared to fetal and maternal sera, suggests a somewhat dynamic exchange of solutes and water between intrauterine compartments. Although fetal urine may well provide the bulk of fluid for this compartment, a low tonicity and apparent high rate of *in utero* urine excretion would suggest that other significant processes are at work to modify the resulting composition and volume of amniotic fluid. The fetus has been reported to swallow approximately 450 ml of amniotic fluid per day.[33] Presumably this fluid and solutes contained therein are reabsorbed by the fetus across the intestinal epithelium. An active sodium pump has been described across fetal intestinal wall,[9] and an obligatory reabsorption of water is also thought to occur. However, such swallowed amniotic fluid would contain a random amount of solute which numerous measurements, even in patients with hydramnios,[19] have shown to fluctuate very little within the usual range of 255-270 mM/liter at term. Therefore, some mechanism must exist for elevating the amniotic fluid solute concentration above that found in fetal urine added to this cavity and for removing a net quantity of fluid from this cavity, since fetal urine is most likely produced in quantities significantly exceeding the amount swallowed by the fetus.

These alterations could in part be accomplished by the diffusion of solutes across membranes separating fetal or maternal compartments from the amniotic fluid, a process favored by the existing steady state gradients, i.e. amniotic fluid hypotonic to maternal and fetal compartments. The net reabsorption of significant quantity of solute-free water from this space should also result from the same gradients, by means of an osmotic transfer of water from the hypotonic amniotic fluid to mother or fetus across any contiguous amniotic and/or chorionic surface. The major difficulties encountered in visualizing such an intrauterine circulation are (1) the relative impermeability of fetal skin to solute and water transfer after keratinization takes place at 24 to 26 weeks, and (2) the absence of a well-developed vascular or capillary bed in apposition to other tissue layers separating intrauterine compartments, such as the chorion laeve and amnion surrounding a major part of the amniotic sac. Thus these tissues present an unlikely site for significant exchange between amniotic sac and maternal or fetal circulation.

Some exchange may take place between the fetal capillary bed in the placenta and the amniotic cavity through the chorionic plate along the posterior placenta, but the diffusion distance is large and little is known about the relative permeability of this tissue. The umbilical cord has been cited as a possible exchange site between fetal circulation and amniotic fluid, but the limited surface area provided by the large vessels within the cord when compared to the effective surface area provided by a capillary network make it a highly unlikely site for significant transfer between the two compartments.

Radio opaque dye introduced into the amniotic cavity from the twelfth week of human pregnancy appeared within the fetal tracheobronchial tree as well as intestinal tract within 18 to 24 hours.[11] The presence of a large capillary network within the fetal lung, along with the comparative hypertonicity of fetal sera to amniotic fluid, suggests that if amniotic fluid is exposed to fetal respiratory tissue in any consistent fashion a net reabsorption of solute-free water should occur from the amniotic space.

However, experimental evidence available indicates that transudation from the nasopharynx and tracheobronchial tree occurs *in utero*.[1, 35] As much as 30 ml/day of isotonic fluid have been estimated to be produced in this fashion. Whether any or all of this fluid is added to the amniotic cavity or whether it is swallowed by the fetus and reabsorbed in the intestine remains unclear.

Although the exact pathway and mechanism of amniotic fluid formation and reabsorption remain obscure, the net addition of 4 to 6 ml of fluid per day from 10 weeks' gestational age until term can be inferred from data on volume and composition changes in this fluid throughout pregnancy. This fluid is isotonic to other maternal and fetal fluids initially, but moderately hypotonic after the fifteenth to twentieth week.

It is quite probable that just as abnormalities in fetal swallowing and urine excretion explain some but not all cases of hydramnios and oligohydramnios, the normal quantities of amniotic fluid swallowed and urine produced by the fetus do not completely account for the net accumulation of amniotic fluid in normal pregnancies. Thus, there are other sources of abnormal and normal fluid production and removal from this cavity. Possible sites include fetal respiratory tract and skin or exchange with fetal and/or maternal compartment across the amnion and chorion either within the placental cake or across the membranes away from the cake. Figure 3-2 indicates known and postulated sites of amniotic fluid formation and removal at term.

ISOTOPIC STUDIES OF INTRAUTERINE FLUID EXCHANGE

Large intrauterine fluid exchanges have been inferred from studies of isotopic water transfer between fetus, mother, and amniotic fluid in humans.[18, 49] The above evidence of fetal urine production and swallowing *in utero,* along with evidence of amniotic fluid production or reaccumulation of excess fluid when this is removed (in acute hydramnios Hutchinson and co-workers have estimated the rate of net reaccumulation in one such case to be about 150 ml/24 hours,[19] and another study[5] suggests that 16-42 ml/hour of amniotic fluid may be produced at term) indicate steady state net exchanges of bulk fluid between these compartments *in utero.* However, the magnitude of such flows in no way approaches the large exchanges inferred from tracer studies, e.g. the turnover or reabsorption of approximately 8 liters/day of amniotic fluid. From previous estimates of very small per diem net increases in this fluid compartment, such tracer data imply similar enormous amniotic fluid production rates.

It is important to emphasize that the transfer of isotopic water between intrauterine compartments in such experiments does not give a quantitative measure of net water movement. The net trans-

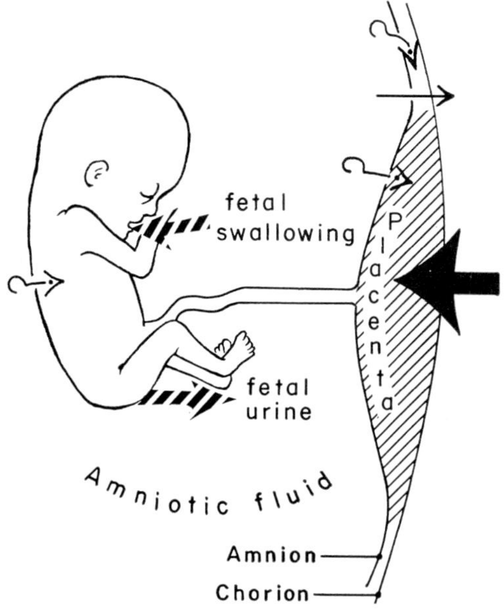

FIGURE 3-2. Known and postulated sites of amniotic fluid formation and removal at term. (From Seeds, A. E.: In Barnes, A. C. (Ed.): *Intra-uterine Development*. Philadelphia, Lea & Febiger, 1968, p. 138.) Early in pregnancy this fluid is probably a dialysate of fetal and maternal extracellular compartments. Recent studies demonstrating significant permeability of fetal skin to isotopic water prior to keratinization at 24 to 26 weeks suggest that this tissue may serve as the site for significant exchange between fetus and amniotic fluid. Later in pregnancy, other exchanges with the fetal circulation provide the major source of amniotic fluid formation and removal. Fetal swallowing and urination do not completely explain the accumulation of moderately hypotonic amniotic fluid over the last half of pregnancy suggesting that the net addition of some solute and reabsorption of solute-free water probably occurs across other tissue layers surrounding this compartment. Possible pathways for exchange with the fetal circulation would include the amnion covering the fetal surface of the placenta and the fetal vessels supplying chorion laeve. Although as much as 30 ml/day of isotonic fluid have been reported to be produced by fetal tracheobronchial and nasopharyngeal secretions, some or all of this fluid may be swallowed, resulting in an unclear picture of the significance of this possible source of amniotic fluid. A small net transfer of water and solute probably takes place from amniotic fluid to maternal extracellular space across the amnion and chorion laeve. The total daily requirements for intrauterine water in pregnancy are most likely provided by a net transfer in response to hydrostatic or osmotic gradients too small or too intermittent to measure.

fer of water or a solvent bulk flow between intrauterine compartments is very difficult to measure by isotopic techniques. For instance, the turnover time of amniotic fluid as measured by the disappearance of tracer water injected into this space is not a measure of a net transfer of water or volume change in this compartment, but an indication of a unidirectional flux of isotopic water in response to a tracer gradient. Most of the isotopic form exchanges on a one-for-one basis, with nonisotopic water across surfaces enclosing the amniotic sac. To measure a net water transfer across a membrane separating two water compartments, the algebraic sum of the two unidirectional water fluxes must be measured. Thus, ideally, a different form of isotopic water should be introduced into each pool and the two unidirectional fluxes computed to measure a net transfer of water. However, because the water concentration is close to 55.6 moles/liter in dilute solutions such as amniotic or other body fluids and most body membranes are very permeable to water, there is always an enormous steady state diffusion flux or exchange of water molecules between contiguous compartments taking place; that is, a one-for-one exchange due to random movements with no volume change in either compartment or net water transfer occurring. Water flux due to random movements will be enormous compared to any net transfer of water due to osmotic or hydrostatic gradients likely to be encountered *in vivo.* Thus measurements of such net transfers by calculation of unidirectional and net fluxes is extremely difficult whether measured by introduction of separate forms of isotopic water into two compartments or calculated by means of elaborate linear compartmental models and analyses.

The apparent large isotopic water exchanges between fetus, amniotic fluid, and maternal compartments in response to a tracer gradient are not an accurate measure of net water transfer in bulk or solvent form between these compartments. However, such studies indicate a very significant *in vivo* permeability to isotopic water across the chorion frondosum and a much smaller exchange per unit gradient across the chorion laeve away from the placental cake, supporting the concept that the highly vascular discoid portion of the placenta is the site of maximum water exchange in pregnancy between maternal and intrauterine compartments.

REGULATION OF AMNIOTIC FLUID VOLUME AND COMPOSITION

Regulation of amniotic fluid volume and composition remains obscure, although it can be surmised empirically that the volume is subject to much wider physiologic and pathologic variation than changes in amniotic fluid total solute concentration. For example, compare the incidence of acute and chronic hydramnios and oligohydramnios as well as the 400 to 1200 ml range in volume considered normal at term to the absence of any disease state known to alter the solute content while the fetus is alive and the apparently very narrow range maintained in total solute concentration throughout pregnancy (Fig. 3-5). Additional experimental evidence of the rather remarkable regulation of amniotic fluid total solute concentration comes from work in the rhesus monkey (Fig. 3-3). Within 18 to 20 hours following replacement of the amniotic fluid with equal volumes of distilled or solute-free water, the total solute concentration had returned to normal or preexperimental levels, accompanied by a significant reduction in volume.[37] In these experiments the normal levels in total solute concentration were reestablished in part by means of a significant reduction in preexisting amniotic fluid volume.

The role of the fetus in regulation of amniotic fluid volume and composition is poorly understood, although most certainly through urine production and swallowing the fetus exerts a large influence on this fluid space and vice versa. There is a high association near term between hydramnios and fetal gastrointestinal or central nervous system anomalies that interfere with swallowing (Table 3-VI), and between oligohydramnios and fetal renal agenesis or dysplasia.[21] There is also an increased incidence of hydramnios associated with the generalized edema of hydrops fetalis encountered in severe erythroblastosis. Experimental work in rabbits indicated a marked reduction in amniotic fluid volume following fetal dehydration.[7] Such findings suggest that amniotic fluid may function as a buffer for fetal water imbalance in that excess water

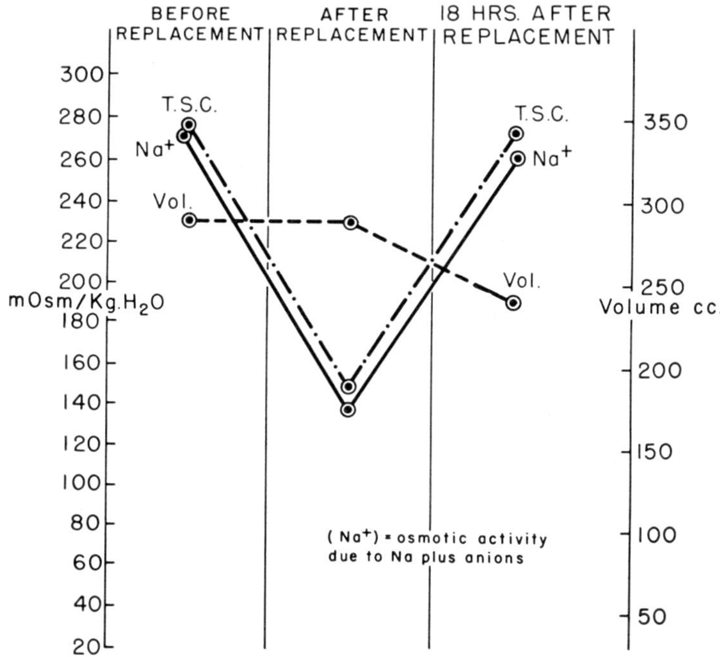

FIGURE 3-3. Eighteen hours following replacement of approximately 25 cc amniotic fluid with an equal volume of distilled water in an experiment with the rhesus monkey, the total solute and sodium concentrations had returned to pre-experimental levels, accompanied by a significant reduction in amniotic fluid volume. Changes in sodium concentration are represented in this figure as osmotic activity due to sodium and corresponding anions. (From Schruefer and co-workers.[37])

accumulation during a period of water intoxication can be excreted into this cavity and water can be extracted from this pool during periods of dehydration. This concept also fits with the overall theory that the amniotic fluid in the latter half of pregnancy is principally a product of the fetal compartment.

CLINICAL SIGNIFICANCE OF AMNIOTIC FLUID

The amniotic fluid compartment may prove to have considerable diagnostic and therapeutic value in the clinical management

TABLE 3-VI

CONGENITAL ANOMALIES ASSOCIATED WITH HYDRAMNIOS*

Anencephaly	32 cases
Iniencephaly	2 "
Hydrops foetalis with gross oedema of the lips and faces	4 "
OEsophageal atresia	12 "
Duodenal atresia	3 "
Diaphragmatic hernia	1 case

*Anomalies occurred in 32% of this series of 169 cases of hydramnios. Table from Jeffcoate, T. N. A., and Scott, J. S.[21]

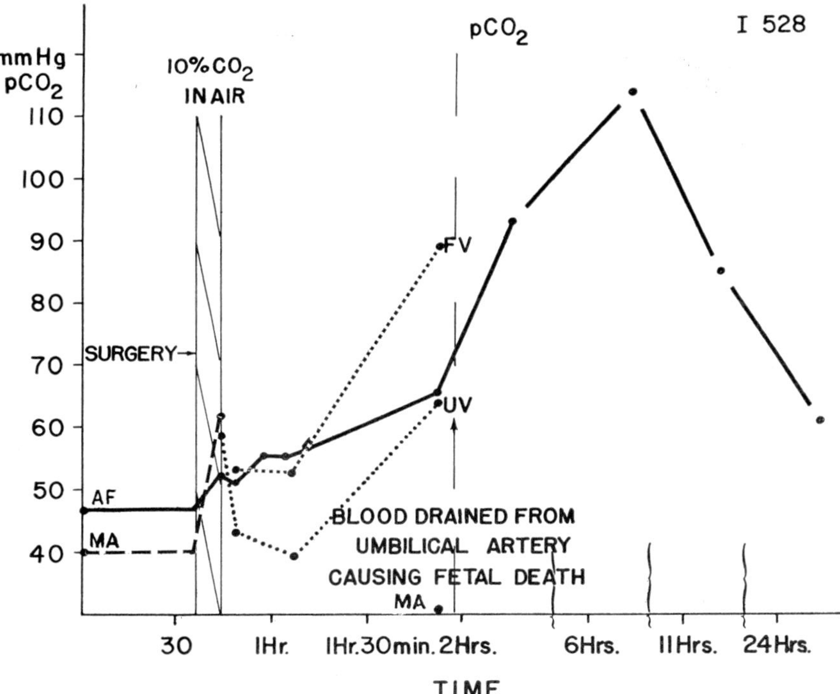

FIGURE 3-4 A, B, C. Changes in (A) PCO_2, (B) pH, and (C) bicarbonate are shown in maternal artery (MA), uterine vein (UV), fetal vein (FV) and amniotic fluid (AF) during and following carbon dioxide administration to the maternal monkey at 130 days' gestation age. Amniotic fluid values were also followed after known fetal death *in utero*. (From Seeds and co-workers.[42])

of the fetus. Recent studies suggest the possibility that this fluid compartment may provide significant information about acute fetal status *in utero* and reflect changes in fetal oxygenation *in utero*. Evidence has also been presented to suggest that infusions into this compartment may be used to medicate the fetus *in utero*. Both concepts gain considerable theoretical support from knowledge that amniotic fluid throughout pregnancy appears to be in large part of fetal origin. To some extent, therefore, chemical changes within one compartment should be reflected in the other.

Work in the rhesus monkey has shown that elevations in fetal plasma carbon dioxide tensions are followed shortly by similar elevations in amniotic fluid P_{CO_2} (Fig. 3-4).[42] Amniotic fluid [HCO_3^-] showed no consistent relationship to fetal bicarbonate content during these experiments. Such data is compatible with previous findings that physically dissolved carbon dioxide rapidly crosses placental tissue while the polar bicarbonate anion diffuses

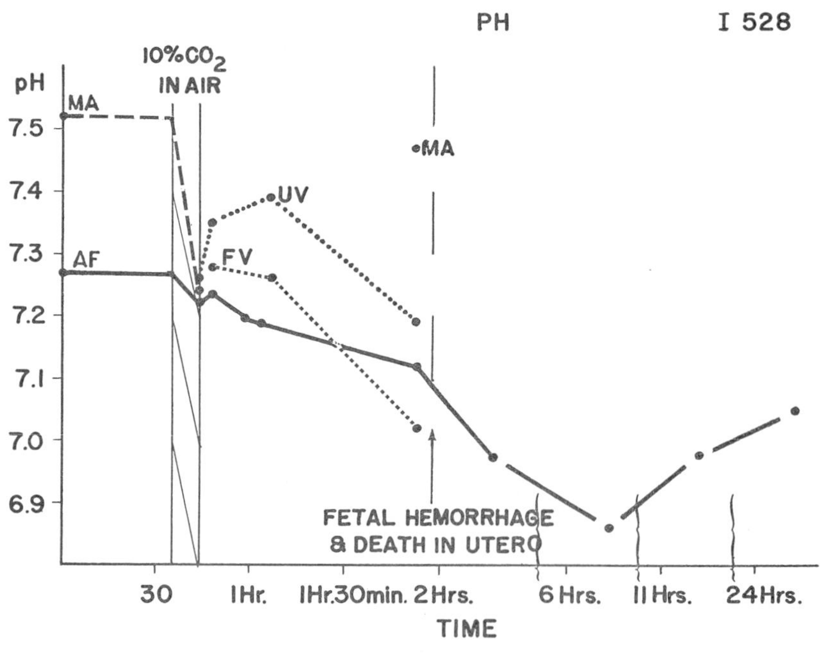

FIGURE 3-4B

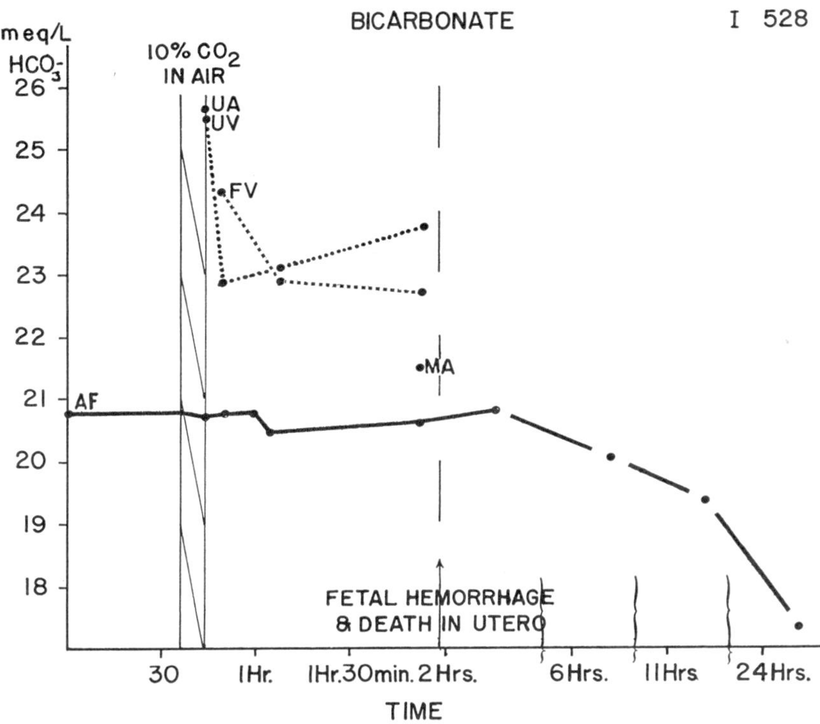

FIGURE 3-4C

only very slowly across these membranes.[6] Fetal hypoxia is almost always accompanied by a "mixed" acidosis wherein the P_{CO_2} is elevated simultaneously with a reduction in bicarbonate content and the severity of the acidosis corresponds to the severity of the hypoxia.[20] Thus it can be expected that a reduction in fetal oxygen supply or fetal distress will be accompanied by a rise in fetal and amniotic fluid P_{CO_2} and a fall in amniotic fluid pH. Confirmation for such a hypothesis comes from the data collected in rhesus monkeys indicating that in all cases of fetal hypercarbia, whether secondary to carbon dioxide administration to the mother or fetal hypoxia, a similar prompt rise in amniotic fluid P_{CO_2} and fall in amniotic fluid pH were observed. Serial measurement of human amniotic fluid indicated that the small decrease in fetal pH during normal labor is accompanied by a corresponding acidotic change in amniotic fluid.[23] Such data suggest the possibility, then, that serial measurement of amniotic fluid acid-base chemistries may provide an indication of fetal acid-base status and oxygenation.

Changes in amniotic fluid acid-base values following fetal death *in utero* were also measured in the monkey (Fig. 3-4). An acute rise in P_{CO_2} followed by a later diminution in amniotic fluid bicarbonate concentration resulted in prolonged reduction in amniotic fluid pH, although the pH appeared to be returning to preexperimental levels within 24 hours after the fetal demise.

Amniotic fluid oxygen tensions apparently do not reflect changes in fetal oxygenation.[46] Steady state amniotic fluid P_{O_2}'s near term in nonlaboring patients have varied between 8 and 25 mm Hg[34, 36 46] and following administration of 100% oxygen to the mother no significant change was noted in the measurements of amniotic fluid P_{O_2} *in vivo*.[46] Technical difficulty with *in vivo* electrode measurements, introduction of blood or an air bubble into the amniotic space during amniocentesis have all been cited as possible causes for the failure of amniotic fluid oxygen measurements to reflect fetal status. However, the most important problem may be that fluctuations in fetal oxygen supply are reflected by changing oxygen concentrations on the steep portion of the fetal oxyhemoglobin dissociation curve. Thus large changes in fetal blood oxygen content are accompanied by relatively small changes in P_{O_2}. Corresponding amniotic fluid P_{O_2} changes are therefore small and difficult to measure during periods of fetal hypoxia.

Data collected in the human suggest that changes in amniotic fluid total solute concentration may reflect fetal status *in utero*[8] (Fig. 3-5). Elevated amniotic fluid total solute concentrations were associated with a much higher incidence of perinatal morbidity and mortality. Although cases of prior fetal death *in utero* showed the most significant increase in total solute concentration, amniocentesis followed by subsequent neonatal death was accompanied by a significant rise in amniotic fluid osmolality. The increased total solute concentration in this series was accompanied by a corresponding elevation in amniotic fluid sodium concentra-

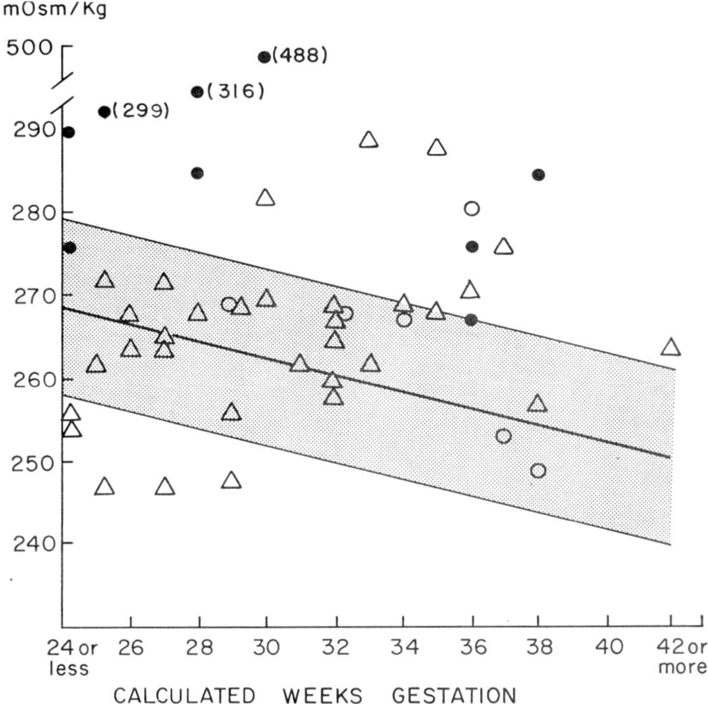

FIGURE 3-5. Relationship between amniotic fluid osmolality (mOsm/kg) and calculated gestational age. Average ± standard error of estimate for 133 amniotic fluids from 83 successful pregnancies with perinatal survival shown as solid line and shaded area (AF osmolality = 288.8-0.90 weeks' gestation; r = -0.30; p = 0.001). Scatterplot points indicate amniotic fluids from 30 unsuccessful pregnancies with prior fetal (solid circles), subsequent fetal (open circles), or subsequent neonatal death (open triangles). (Consecutive samples collected within 24 hrs of each other are averaged and indicated as single points-6 such fluids are represented by 3 points in this figure.) (From Cassady, G., and Barnett, R.[8])

tion. Such findings are consistent with previously discussed evidence of a marked increase in fetal urine total solute concentration during periods of stress.[3]

Experiments in the rhesus monkey have shown that the fetal pH can be elevated by means of amniotic fluid infusions of sodium bicarbonate.[40] Elevations in fetal plasma bicarbonate, buffer base, and pH (in one case to 7.60) were observed in these animals.

Simultaneous measurement of fetal plasma osmolality showed no significant change, indicating that this net increase in fetal bicarbonate was not associated with plasma hypertonicity, but apparently resulted from an exchange of bicarbonate for chloride. These findings might be expected if most of the fetal bicarbonate accumulation was secondary to swallowing of the very alkaline amniotic fluid and absorption of bicarbonate across intestinal mucosa. Although such a mechanism may in part explain fetal alkalinization during these experiments, other exchange sites between fetus and amniotic fluid should also be considered. Thus the introduction of 40 to 80 mEq $NaHCO_3$ into the amniotic cavity created an enormous gradient in chemical potential favoring the diffusion of bicarbonate into the fetal compartment across any contiguous, permeable membrane.

The specific value of amniotic fluid bicarbonate infusions remains ambiguous. Although parenteral bicarbonate infusions are used by some clinicians to treat the acidosis accompanying hypoxia in the newborn, the primary deficit remains the oxygen supply to the fetus. That is, at the very low *in utero* oxygen tensions found during hypoxia, it is questionable what benefit even a pronounced increase in fetal pH would have. Current studies in animals[17, 43] wherein fetal pH is experimentally manipulated up or down show little change in fetal oxygen content or consumption, but only fluctuations in fetal Po_2 as if in response to a new position of the fetal oxyhemoglobin dissociation curve. Thus, instead of increasing fetal oxygen concentration or supply, fetal pH changes simply repartitioned the available oxygen between that bound to hemoglobin and the small fraction dissolved in plasma water. Nevertheless, the amniotic fluid bicarbonate infusions represent an interesting experimental model wherein a pharmacologic substance was introduced into the fetus *in utero* by means of amniotic fluid infusions.

REFERENCES

1. Adams, F.H., Fujiwara, T., and Rowshan, G.: The nature and origin of the fluid in the fetal lamb lung. *J Pediatr, 63:*881, 1963.
2. Alexander, D.P., and Nixon, D.A.: The fœtal kidney. *Br Med Bull, 17:* 112, 1961.

3. Alexander, D.P., Nixon, D.A., Widdas, W.F., and Wahlzogen, F.X.: Renal function in the sheep fetus. *J Physiol, 140:*14, 1958.
4. Battaglia, F.C., Prystowsky, H., Smisson, C., Hellegers, A.E., and Bruns, P.D.: Fetal blood studies XVI. On the changes in total osmotic pressure and sodium and potassium concentrations of amniotic fluid during the course of human gestation. *Surg Gynecol Obstet, 109:*509, 1959.
5. Biggs, J.S., Duncan, R.O.: Production rate and sources of amniotic fluid at term. *J Obstet Gynaecol Br Commonw, 77:*326, 1970.
6. Blechner, J.N., Meschia, G., and Barron, D.H.: A study of the acid-base balance of fetal sheep and goats. *Q J Exp Physiol, 45:*60, 1960.
7. Bruns, P.D., Linder, R.O., Drose, V.E., and Battaglia, F.C.: The placental transfer of water from fetus to mother following the intravenous infusion of hypertonic mannitol to the maternal rabit. *Am J Obstet Gynecol, 86:*160, 1963.
8. Cassady, G., and Barnett, R.: Amniotic fluid electrolytes and perinatal outcome. *Biol Neonate, 13:*155, 1968.
9. Chez, R.A.: Ion transport by the primate neonatal stomach. *Invest Gynecol, 1:*39, 1970.
10. Chez, R.A., Smith, F.G., and Hutchinson, D.L.: Renal function in the intrauterine primate fetus. *Am J Obstet Gynecol, 90:*128, 1964.
11. Davis, M.E., and Potter, E.L.: Intrauterine respiration of the human fetus. *JAMA, 131:*1194, 1961.
12. Dowd, P.M., Rudge, P.J., and Harris, J.W.S.: The volume of amniotic fluid in the first half of pregnancy. *J Anat, 105:*207, 1969.
13. Elliott, P.M., and Inman, W.H.W.: Volume of liquor amnii in normal and abnormal pregnancy. *Lancet, 2:*835, 1961.
14. Gadd, R.L.: The volume of liquor amnii in normal and abnormal pregnancies. *J Obstet Gynaecol Br Commonw, 73:*11, 1966.
15. Gillebrand, P.N.: Changes in amniotic fluid volume with advancing pregnancy. *J Obstet Gynaecol Br Commonw, 76:*527, 1969.
16. Harrison, R.G., and Malpas, P.: The volume of human amniotic fluid. *J Obstet Gynaecol Br Commonw, 60:*632, 1953.
17. Hellegers, A.E., Armstead, E.E., Thomas, C.E., Burnett, A.M., MacGovern, T.J., and Bruns, P.D.: Effect of fetal metabolic acidosis upon oxygen environment. *Am J Obstet Gynecol, 105:*786, 1969.
18. Hutchinson, D.L., Gray, M.J., Plentl, A.A., Alvarez, H., Caldeyro-Barcia, R., Kaplan, B., and Lind, J.: The role of the fetus in the water exchange of the amniotic fluid of normal and hydramniotic patients. *J Clin Invest, 38:*971, 1959.
19. Hutchinson, D.L., Hunter, C.B., Neslen, E.D., and Plentl, A.A.: The exchange of water and electrolytes in the mechanism of amniotic fluid formation and the relationship to hydramnios. *Surg Gynecol Obstet 100:* 391, 1955.
20. James, L.S., Weisbrot, I.M., Prince, C.E., Holoday, D.A., and Apgar, V.:

The acid-base status of human infants in relation to birth asphyxia and the onset of respiration. *J Pediatr, 52:*379, 1958.

21. Jeffcoate, T.N.A., and Scott, J.S.: Polyhydramnios and oligohydramnios. *Can Med Assoc J, 80:*77, 1959.
22. Kerr, G.R., and Kennan, A.L.: The free amino acids of amniotic fluid during pregnancy of the rhesus monkey. *Am J Obstet Gynecol, 105:*363, 1969.
23. Kittrich, M.: Changes in acid-base balance of amniotic fluid during labor. *J Obstet Gynaecol Br Commonw, 75:*1138, 1968.
24. Makepiece, A.W., Fremont-Smith, F., Dailey, M.E., and Carroll, M.P.: The nature of the amniotic fluid. A comparative study of human amniotic fluid and maternal serum. *Surg Gynecol Obstet, 53:*635, 1931.
25. McCance, R.A., and Widdowson, E.M.: Renal function before birth. *Proc R Soc Lond* (Biol), *141:*488, 1953.
26. McCance, R.A., and Widdowson, E.M.: Renal aspects of acid-base control in the newly born. 1. Natural development. *Acta Paediatr 49:*409, 1960.
27. McClure Browne, J.C.: Postmaturity. *Am J Obstet Gynecol, 85:*573, 1963.
28. McGaughey, H.S., Carey, E.L., Scoggin, W.A., Bobbitt, O.B., and Thornton, N.M.: Observations on the equilibration of urea between baby and mother at term. *Am J Obstet Gynecol, 78:*845, 1959.
29. McGaughey, H.S., Carey, E.L., Scoggin, W.A., Ficklen, G.H., and Thornton, N.M.: Creatinine transport between baby and mother at term. *Am J Obstet Gynecol, 80:*108, 1960.
30. Monie, I.W.: The volume of the amniotic fluid in the early months of pregnancy. *Am J Obstet Gynecol, 66:*616, 1953.
31. Moya, F., Apgar, V., James, L.S., and Berrieu, C.: Hydramnios and congenital anomalies. Study of series of seventy-four patients. *JAMA, 173:* 1552, 1960.
32. Parmley, T., and Seeds, A.E.: Permeability of fetal skin to tritiated water. *Am J Obstet Gynecol, 108:*128, 1970.
33. Pritchard, J.A.: Deglutition by normal and anencephalic fetuses. *Obstet Gynecol 25:*289, 1965.
34. Quilligan, E.J.: Amniotic fluid gas tensions. *Am J Obstet Gynecol, 84:* 20, 1962.
35. Reynolds, S.R.M.: A source of amniotic fluid in the lamb: The nasopharyngeal and buccal cavities. *Nature, 172:*307, 1953.
36. Romney, S.L., Kaneoka, T., Gabel, P.V.: Perinatal oxygen environment. Polarigraphic determinations of oxygen tension in umbilical cord blood and amniotic fluid of normal term newborn infants. *Am J Obstet Gynecol, 84:*25, 1962.
37. Schruefer, J.J.P., Seeds, A.E., Battaglia, F.C., Hellegers, A.E., Behrman, R.E., Bruns, P.D.: Changes in amniotic fluid volume and total solute

concentration in the rhesus monkey following replacement with distilled water. Measurement of amniotic fluid volume by I^{131} albumin dilution. (in press) *Am J Obstet Gynecol.*

38. Seeds, A.E.: Water metabolism of the fetus. *Am J Obstet Gynecol, 92:*727, 1965.
39. Seeds, A.E., Behrman, R.E., Battaglia, F.C., Hellegers, A.E., and Bruns, P.D.: Changes in amniotic fluid total solute concentrations in the rhesus monkey. *Am J Obstet Gynecol, 89:*476, 1964.
40. Seeds, A.E., Bissonnette, J.M., Lim, H., and Behrman, R.E.: Changes in rhesus monkey fetal and maternal acid-base measurements following amniotic fluid bicarbonate or Tris infusions. *Am J Obstet Gynecol, 107:*232, 1970.
41. Seeds, A.E., and Hellegers, A.E.: Acid-base determinations in human amniotic fluid throughout pregnancy. *Am J Obstet Gynecol, 101:*257, 1968.
42. Seeds, A.E., Kock, H.C., Myers, R.C., Stolte, L.A.M., and Hellegers, A.E.: Changes in rhesus monkey amniotic fluid pH, pCO_2, and bicarbonate concentration following maternal and fetal hypercarbia and fetal death in utero. *Am J Obstet Gynecol, 97:*67, 1967.
43. Seeds, A.E., Schruefer, J.J.P., Parmley, T., Hellegers, A.E., Lim, H.S., and Simkovich, J.: Unpublished data.
44. Sinha, R., and Carlton, M.: The volume and composition of amniotic fluid in early pregnancy. *J Obstet Gynaecol Br Commonw, 77:*211, 1970.
45. Smith, F.G., Adams, F.H., Borden, M., and Hilburn, J.: Studies of renal function in the intact fetal lamb. *Am J Obstet Gynecol, 96:*240, 1966.
46. Vasicka, A.: Oxygen in the amniotic fluid. *Clin Obstet Gynecol, 9:*461, 1966.
47. Von Friedberg, V.: Untersuchungan uber die fetale Urinbildung. *Gynaecologia, 140:*34, 1955.
48. Vonnegut, F.A.: Systematische Fruchtwassermessungen in den verschiedenen Schwangerschaftsmonaten. *Zentralbl Gynaekol, 52:*1306, 1928.
49. Vosburgh, G.J., Flexner, L.B., Courie, D.B., Hellman, L.M., Proctor, N.K., and Wilde, W.S.: The rate of renewal in women of the water and sodium of the amniotic fluid as determined by tracer gradients. *Am J Obstet Gynecol, 56:*1156, 1948.
50. Wagner, G., and Fuchs, F.: The volume of amniotic fluid in the first half of human pregnancy. *J Obstet Gynaecol Br Commonw, 69:*131, 1962.
51. Wood, C.: Weightlessness: Its implications for the human fetus. *J Obstet Gynaecol Br Commonw, 77:*333, 1970.
52. Woolf, L.I., and Norman, A.P.: The urinary excretion of amino acids and sugars in early infancy. *J Pediatr, 50:*271, 1957.
53. Yordan, E., D'Esopo, A.D.: Hydramnios. A review of 204 cases at the Sloan Hospital for Women. *Am J Obstet Gynecol, 70:*266, 1955.

Chapter 4

TECHNIQUE OF AMNIOCENTESIS

Allan C. Barnes

There are in general three motivations for transabdominal amniocentesis:

1. To administer hypertonic saline in therapeutic pregnancy termination.

2. To obtain amniotic fluid for intrauterine diagnostic procedure.

3. To insert a catheter for the chronic monitoring of intrauterine pressures and pressure changes.

As indicated below, there may be minor variations in the procedure, depending on which of these indications may apply, but, in all circumstances, sterile technique is imperative. Whether the uterus is to be evacuated or the pregnancy preserved, amnionitis and endometritis represent grave threats to the mother.

Accordingly, the abdomen should be as well prepared as for any surgery procedure, including shaving, where necessary.

The bladder should be empty, although there is no clear evidence that the needle passing in and out of the bladder on its way to the uterine cavity will produce any serious difficulties.

The best location for an initial attempt to enter the amniotic cavity is in the midline immediately suprapubicly. The needle (14 gauge, 4 inch) should be angled 30 degrees cephalad, or approximately toward the promontory of the sacrum. After the needle has passed through the skin, the trochar should be removed, a syringe attached, and the needle advanced further with gentle suction applied. If a free flow of blood is encountered, this means under most circumstances that the needle has intravillous space. If the pregnancy is to be preserved (i.e. the tap is purely for diagnostic reasons), the needle should be withdrawn and an attempt made in another location. It must be stressed that there is no evidence that fetal damage or that fetal hazard will occur from the mere perforation of the maternal surface of the placenta. Conversely, the fetus is put at a definite risk if the fetal plate of the placenta is violated.

If the indications for amniocentesis are for the administration of saline, the needle can continue to be advanced with a gentle suction, despite encountering blood. When amniotic fluid is obtained, the syringe should be changed so that one can accurately evaluate the amount of hemoglobin contaminating the fluid itself. A slightly blood-tinged fluid is not a contraindication to the administration of saline, whereas heavily contaminated fluid, which might indicate an open vessel, would be considered a contraindication.

Very often up to 5 cc of fluid can be obtained as early as the 14th week, but 10 cc can rarely be obtained prior to the 16th week. The handling of the fluid in diagnostic cases would be dependent on which studies were contemplated although, under all circumstances, it is good to keep the fluid away from exposure to light.

Almost as a portion of the technique involved, it should be pointed out that if the diagnostic determination is a simple one (i.e. determining the gender of the fetus in sex-linked diseases), the operative permit for pregnancy interruption should be signed before amniocentesis is carried out. Very often (and preferably) the instillation of saline can be carried out on the same hospital day. This not only could reduce hospitalization, but potentially reduces any hours of discussion and indecision. Certainly there is no need to carry out the diagnostic studies if the appropriate therapy is to be refused by the patient.

A few additional precautions should be taken when performing amniocentesis later in pregnancy to minimize the possibility of injury to the placenta. The fetal position should be palpated and the placental souffle should be localized if possible. Assuming the fetal presentation (usually vertex) can be determined abdominally, the amniotic sac can usually be entered without difficulty at a site away from the body of the fetus where fluid is most likely to be found. This area frequently is somewhere between the umbilicus and symphysis, close to the midline. Since the placenta is more likely to be implanted on the upper rather than lower portion of the uterus, the chance of trauma to this organ is reduced by favoring the lower abdominal route for amniocentesis, particularly when placental localization is difficult. As previously described, the needle should be carefully advanced through the uterine wall and a free flow of blood should result in immediate withdrawal and selection of another site for the procedure. A history of previous abdominal surgery or severe pelvic infection should also alert the operator to the possibility of adherent loops of bowel on the anterior surface of the uterus or abdominal wall.

Chapter 5

BIOCHEMICAL AND CYTOLOGIC COMPONENTS OF AMNIOTIC FLUID

HENRY L. NADLER

Amniotic fluid has been used with increasing frequency for intrauterine diagnosis. In the vast majority of cases, amniotic fluid obtained by transabdominal amniocentesis has been utilized for the management of Rh iso-immunization, assessment of fetal maturity or assessment of fetal jeopardy. More recently, amniotic fluid has been utilized for the *in utero* detection of genetic disorders. The present state of knowledge of the cytologic and biochemical properties of amniotic fluid as pertains to the *in utero* detection of genetic defects (excluding Rh iso-immunization) and the estimation of gestational age will be reviewed.

Amniotic fluid is composed of 98% to 99% water with 1% to 2% solids. The inorganic constituents of amniotic fluid are quite similar to extracellular fluid, and the solids are equally divided between organic solids and proteins. Excellent reviews of the composition of amniotic fluid have recently been published.[1, 2]

BIOCHEMICAL COMPONENTS OF AMNIOTIC FLUID

Gases

The concentration of respiratory gases in the amniotic fluid has been studied by many investigators and is discussed in another chapter of this book. Suffice it to say that the concentration of respiratory gases in amniotic fluid in association with amniotic fluid pH may provide useful information regarding fetal jeopardy shortly prior to and during delivery.

Electrolytes

The amniotic fluid prior to 20 weeks of pregnancy is thought to represent a dialysate of maternal serum based upon the finding that the concentration of electrolytes is essentially that found in maternal serum.[3-5] During the latter half of pregnancy, the amniotic fluid becomes increasingly hypotonic. Although electrolyte concentrations have been studied, no directly defined relationship between fetal or maternal jeopardy has been established.

Proteins and Protein Derivatives

The proteins of amniotic fluid have been investigated and although considerable variation has been found, useful ranges have been established.[4, 6, 7] The amino acid composition of amniotic fluid has been studied and quantitated both late in pregnancy[8-12] and more recently, early in pregnancy.[13] Emery et al.[13] have quantitated the amino acid composition of amniotic fluid from the 9th week of gestation to term. Although serial studies were not performed, this information should prove useful for the antenatal diagnosis of certain genetic disorders. Morrow et al.[14] have recently detected methylmalonic acidemia in a fetus by observing increasing amounts of methylmalonic acid in amniotic fluid and maternal urine during the third trimester of pregnancy.

The origin of all proteins in amniotic fluid is not firmly established. Conflicting reports have suggested the proteins are of maternal origin[15, 16] while others[17, 18] present evidence attempting to show their fetal origin. Other nitrogenous constituents such as amniotic fluid urea, uric acid, and creatinine increase late in pregnancy and at term are approximately twice that found in maternal serum.[4, 7, 19] The potential usefulness of this finding will be discussed in the section on estimation of gestational age.

Knowledge of the protein components of amniotic fluid may be useful as markers of genetic disorders possibly through linkage analysis. Marks et al.[19] have suggested that the antenatal detection of X-linked uricaciduria (Lesch-Nyhan Syndrome) might be detected on the basis of increased amniotic fluid uric acid levels.

Hormones

The following hormones have been reported as being present in amniotic fluid: cortisol,[20] cortisone,[20] pregnanetriol,[21, 22] pregnanediol,[23] progesterone,[1] 17-hydroxycorticosteroids,[24, 25] 17-ketosteroids,[21, 22, 26] estrone, estradiol and estriol,[27-31] chorionic gonadotropin[32] and placental lactogen.[33]

Jeffcoate and associates,[21] Fuchs[34] and Nichols[35] have been able to establish the antenatal diagnosis of the adrenogenital syndrome by measuring the levels of 17-ketosteroids and pregnanetriol in amniotic fluid late in pregnancy. Merkatz et al.[22] were unable to predict this disorder during early or middle pregnancy using levels of 17-ketosteroids or pregnanetriol despite their suggestive elevations in amniotic fluid obtained at term from affected pregnancies.

Enzymes

A number of enzymes have been detected in amniotic fluid; however, in some instances it is impossible to determine whether the enzymes detected were, in fact, found in the amniotic fluid supernatant or in the amniotic fluid cells. These enzymes have been detected in amniotic fluid: α-glucosidase,[36] acid phosphatase,[37-39] aldolase,[40, 41] alanine transaminase,[42, 43] alkaline phosphatase,[37-39] aminotripeptidase,[1] amylase,[42, 43] aspartate transaminase,[42, 43] β-glucuronidase,[44] carboxypeptidase,[1] cathepsin,[37] cholinesterase,[45] diamine oxidase,[46, 47] diastase,[48] glutamic oxalacetic transaminase,[40, 49, 50] glutamic pyruvic transaminase,[40,50] hexoseaminidoses A and B[85, 86] histaminase,[51] kininogen,[52] lactate dehydrogenase,[40, 41, 49] leucine aminopeptidase,[53, 54] lipase,[48] lysozyme,[55] malic dehydrogenase,[40] monomine oxidase,[56, 57] p-phenylenediamine oxidase,[58] pepsinogen,[48, 37] phosphohexoisomerase,[1] and ribose-5-PO_4 isomerase.[1]

Nadler and Messina[36] have reported a deficiency of α-glucosidase activity in amniotic fluid when the fetus was affected with Pompe's disease. On this basis they have suggested that levels of amniotic fluid α-glucosidase might be useful in the antenatal detection of this disorder. More recently, Nadler et al.[59] have failed to confirm this observation in another case in which the *in utero* diagnosis of Pompe's disease was established. These observations suggest that direct analysis of amniotic fluid may not be a reliable method for the intrauterine diagnosis of other familial metabolic disorders. Potential sources of error include the presence of maternal isoenzymes and fetal enzymes.

Other Components

Amniotic fluid levels of sugars, lipids, bilirubin, protein-bound iodine, and other components have been reviewed[1, 2] and will be discussed only in relationship to estimates of fetal age.

Matalon et al.[60] have recently reported the antenatal detection of mucopolysaccharidosis based upon the quantitative and qualitative changes of mucopolysaccharides found in amniotic fluid.

AMNIOTIC FLUID CELLS

The utilization of the cellular material found in amniotic fluid, which has been shown to be derived from amnion and fetus[61, 62] initially focused upon the technique of sex chromatin analysis for the antenatal determination of sex.[63-71, 99] The presence of sex chromatin in amniotic fluid cells has been useful for the management of pregnancies in women heterozygous for X-linked recessive disorders such as hemophilia and muscular dystrophy.[72-74] However, accurate diagnosis is not possible in all cases[99] and chromosome analysis on cultivated amniotic fluid cells should be utilized to determine the sex of the fetus.

Fuchs and associates[75] and others[76, 77] have been able to demonstrate immunogenetic markers in desquamated amniotic fluid cells. Gordon and Brosens[78] have reported a direct relationship between fetal age and the ability of the desquamated cells to stain orange with Nile blue sulfate. This will be discussed in the section concerning assessment of fetal maturity.

Electron microscopic studies of uncultured amniotic fluid cells have been utilized to establish the antenatal diagnosis of Pompe's disease.[79] Abnormal membrane-surrounded lysosomes could be detected in uncultured cells[79] as well as cultivated cells.[59]

Biochemical studies of uncultured amniotic fluid cells have shown the following enzymes to be detectable: α-glucosidase,[36, 80] aryl sulfatase,[81] adenylate pyrophosphate phosphoribosyl transferase,[82] acid phosphatase,[83] alkaline phosphatase,[83] arginase,[83] β-galactosidase,[81] β-glucuronidase,[83] β-D-N-acetylglucosaminidase,[81] galactose-1-phosphate uridyl transferase,[83] glucose-6-phosphate dehydrogenase,[83, 84] hexoseaminidases A and B,[85, 86] hypoxanthine guanine phosphoribosyl transferase,[82] isocitrate dehydrogenase,[84] lactate dehydrogenase,[83, 84] ornithine transcarbamylase,[83] 6-phosphogluconic dehydrogenase,[83, 84] phosphohexose isomerase,[84] and valine transaminase.[87]

The normal ranges of enzyme activities in uncultured amniotic fluid cells must be adequately defined before they become useful for antenatal detection of genetic disorders. The antenatal detection of Pompe's disease[36] and Tay-Sachs disease[88] has been established utilizing uncultured amniotic fluid cells. Great caution should be taken when attempting to use amniotic fluid cells directly for enzyme analysis. Rattazzi and Davidson[86] have shown that hexosaminidase A is unstable in noncultured cells, hence a demonstration of the deficiency of this enzyme in uncultured amniotic fluid cells may be unreliable.

CULTIVATED AMNIOTIC FLUID CELLS

Recently a number of investigators have demonstrated the ability to culture amniotic fluid cells.[89-99, 105] Successful cultivation has been achieved with increasing frequency. In a number of large series, the rates of successful cultivation of amniotic fluid cells for chromosome analysis approaches 97 percent on a single sample of amniotic fluid.[74, 100] The rates of successful cultivation of amniotic fluid in the same hands through a number of subcultures falls to approximately 80 percent. The methods used to cultivate amniotic fluid differ significantly from one another and success rates do not appear to be dependent upon any specific factors with the possible exception of experience and care in handling cells.

Chromosome analysis of cultivated amniotic fluid obtained by transabdominal amniocentesis between the 12th and 20th week of pregnancy has been utilized to manage over 300 pregnancies at risk for cytogenetic aberrations.[74, 100, 101] The indications for study in this group included chromosomal translocation carriers, maternal age greater than 40 years, previous trisomic Down's syndrome and carriers of X-linked recessive disorders. The intrauterine diagnosis of Down's syndrome, either trisomic or translocation forms, has been established in 16 cases[74, 101-103, 119] and in 15 instances the pregnancy was terminated.

Chromosome analysis has been accurate in all but three of over 300 cases.[74, 104] The errors in these cases were presumably caused by the inadvertent growth of maternal cells. This complication could be reduced in frequency if chromosome analysis is performed on duplicate cultures at least 10 days after initiation of the culture. At the present time, based upon the experience with chromosome analysis of amniotic fluid cells, the procedure would appear to be clinically useful and practical in the management of high risk cytogenetic pregnancies.

Biochemical studies of cultivated amniotic fluid cells have been reported by a number of investigators. The enzymes listed below have been detected in cultivated amniotic fluid cells obtained early in pregnancy: acid phosphatase,[105] alkaline phosphatase,[105] α-glucosidase,[36, 80, 105] α-keto-isocaproate decarboxylase,[104, 106, 119] amylo-1, 6-glucosidase,[142] argininosuccinase,[107] aryl sulfatase,[74, 81] β-galactosidase,[74, 108] β-D-N-acetylglucosaminidase,[81] β-glucosidase,[109] β-glucuronidase,[105] cystathionine synthase,[110] galactose-1-phosphate uridyl transferase,[105] glucocerebrosidase,[119] glucose-6-phosphate dehydrogenase,[105] hexoseaminidase A and B,[86, 111] hypoxanthine guanine phosphoribosyl transferase,[112, 113] lactate dehydrogenase,[105] phytanic acid α-hydroxylase,[119] 6-phosphogluconic dehydrogenase,[105] sphingomyelinase,[119] sulfatide sulfatase,[104] valine transminase.[87]

The intracellular distribution of glucose-6-phosphate dehydrogenase, lactate dehydrogenase, acid phosphatase, α-glucosidase and β-glucuronidase in cultivated amniotic fluid cells is similar to their distribution in fibroblasts derived from skin biopsies of children and adults. Kaback et al.[114] have reported significant differences in the specific activity of β-galactosidase, β-D-N-acetylglucosaminidase and aryl sulfatase A in fetal skin, cultured amniotic fluid cells and maternal skin. The normal developmental pattern and distribution for each enzyme derived from amniotic fluid cells should be known before attempting to utilize the information for intrauterine diagnosis. Qualitative changes of lactate dehydrogenase and glucose-6-phosphate dehydrogenase in cultivated amniotic fluid cells obtained early in pregnancy have been reported.[105]

The antenatal detection of a number of familial metabolic disorders utilizing cultivated amniotic fluid cells has been reported.[36, 59, 74, 113, 115-118] The disorders detected *in utero* include X-linked uric aciduria,[113] galactosemia,[115] lysosomal acid phosphatase deficiency,[118] mucopolysaccharidosis,[115, 116] Pompe's disease,[36, 59, 79, 80] cystic fibrosis,[117] and metachromatic leukodystrophy.[74] The pregnancies were terminated and the diagnosis confirmed using abortion material. In other cases, pregnancies at risk for producing a fetus with a genetic defect have been monitored and normal children, some of whom were carriers, were delivered.[74, 104, 112, 121] In some cases, diagnosis appears to be accurate and reliable; in others, cystic fibrosis for example, the methods of detection lack precision and reliability and therefore cannot be used for intrauterine diagnosis. A great deal more experience is required before cultivated amniotic fluid cells can be used as a routine method for the antenatal detection of familial metabolic disorders.

ESTIMATION OF FETAL MATURITY

The accurate assessment of fetal maturity is a prerequisite for the management of many conditions resulting in fetal jeopardy. The problem of optimal time of delivery in cases of diabetes, toxemia, iso-immunization, postmaturity and repeat cesarean sections is complex. One must weigh the advantages of early delivery against the risks of prematurity. Although there have been many attempts at assessment of fetal maturity including past menstrual history, physical examination, ultrasonics and x-ray, this discussion will concern itself with the potential usefulness of amniotic fluid to estimate gestational age. An excellent review of amniotic fluid studies for determination of fetal maturity has recently been published by Andrews.[122]

Bilirubin levels in amniotic fluid have been utilized by a number of investigators.[123-126] This method utilizes the spectrophotometric analysis of amniotic fluid for bilirubin in the manner described by Liley.[127] Mandelbaum, La Croix and Robinson[123] reported the finding of a precipitous fall of the amniotic fluid absorbance bulge at 450 mμ at 36 to 38 weeks' gestation in unsensitized pregnancies. In this series, the absence of spectrophotometric absorbance at 450 mμ was always associated with the birth of an infant weighing more than 5 pounds. In the series of Wiser and Thiede,[126] only 7 of 42 samples obtained at 38 weeks or later had changes in optical density greater than 0.01. This was in contrast to the data on samples obtained prior to 38 weeks when 24 of 48 demonstrated differences greater than 0.01. White and co-workers[125] reported the finding of changes in optical density significantly greater than 0.01 after 38 weeks in nonsensitized patients. These cases were women with diabetes and toxemia who delivered infants less than 2500 grams.

Amniotic fluid creatinine has been suggested as a reliable indicator of fetal maturity.[128-130] The concentration of creatinine increases from 32 to 36 weeks gestation and a value of 2 mg% was indicative of maturity in 95 percent of the cases in a number of series.[129, 130] In another study, values greater than 1.5 mg% were always associated with the birth of an infant weighing more than 2500 grams. In contrast, Wiser and Thiede[126] found values greater than 2 mg% in only 31 percent of the cases while Andrews[122] reports the finding of levels above 2 mg% in 10 percent of the infants below 36 weeks' gestation.

Amniotic fluid osmolality has been suggested as another method for estimating fetal maturity.[131, 132] An amniotic fluid osmolality level of 250 mOsm/liter or less has been suggested as indicating fetal maturity.[131] Uric acid levels in amniotic fluid have been found to be elevated late in pregnancy and might possibly be of value.

Examination of desquamated amniotic fluid cells has been suggested as another method for assessment of fetal maturity.[133-137] Brosens and Gordon[134, 136] applied the technique of staining amniotic fluid cells with Nile blue sulfate, as previously reported by Kittrich,[133] in an attempt to estimate fetal maturity. A marked increase in orange staining cells was seen after 36 weeks' gestation. No premature infants were delivered when more than 20 percent of the amniotic fluid cells stained orange in the series of Bishop and Corson.[137] The question of whether the lipid material which stains orange is intracellular or extracellular has not been resolved.

Most recently, the changes in phospholipids in amniotic fluid have been utilized for estimating maturity.[138-140] Intuitively this approach is the most promising as it provides a method which permits prediction of the outcome of the pregnancy as well as assessing fetal maturity. The assessment of pulmonary maturity of the fetus is most important as respiratory distress syndrome is a major cause of death in the premature infant. The chemical character of phospholipids in amniotic fluid suggests that they have arisen largely in the fetal lung[141] and that they could provide a method of accurate assessment of pulmonary maturity. Gluck et al.[140] have reported the largest series in which changes in amniotic fluid phospholipids have been shown to reflect the changes in the lung of the developing fetus. They were able to relate the rapid increase in lecithin concentration occurring after 35 weeks' gestation to maturity of the fetal lung. They have suggested a screening test in which the appearance of a lecithin spot larger than that of sphingomyelin on thin layer silica gel could be interpreted as indicating pulmonary maturity in the fetus.

Estimates of fetal maturity should be based upon a number of these and possibly other tests rather than on any single measurement. It is quite probable that reliable interpretation of amniotic fluid samples may require serial determinations in order to assess the particular patterns of change that evolve.

REFERENCES

1. Bonsnes,R.W.: Composition of amniotic fluid. *Clin Obstet Gynecol, 9:*440, 1966.
2. Ostergard, D.R.: The physiology and clinical importance of amniotic fluid. A review. *Obstet Gynecol Survey, 25:*297, 1970.
3. Tankard, A.R., Bagnall, D.S.T., and Morris, F.: The composition of amniotic fluid. *Analyst, 59:*806, 1934.

4. Barnes, A.C. (Ed.): *Intrauterine Development.* Philadelphia, Lea and Febiger, 1968.
5. Behrman, R.E., Parer, J.T., and de Lannoy, C.W., Jr.: Placental growth and the formation of amniotic fluid. *Nature, 214:*678, 1967.
6. Abbas, T.M., and Tovey, J.E.: Proteins of the liquor amnii. *Br Med J, 1:*476, 1960.
7. Shrewsbury, J.F.D.: Observations of the chemistry of liquor amnii. *Lancet, 1:*415, 1933.
8. Orlandi, C., Torsello, R.V., and Bottiglioni, F.: Analisi qualitativa e dosaggio semiquantitativo degli aminoacidi contenuti nel liquido amniotico. *Attual Ostet Ginecol, 4:*871, 1958.
9. Wirtschafter, Z.T.: Free amnio acids in human amniotic fluid, fetal and maternal serum. *Am J Obstet Gynecol, 76:*1219, 1958.
10. Sassi, D.: Sulla presenza degli aminoacidi nel liquido amniotico. *Monogr Ostet Ginecol, 33:*683, 1962.
11. Spackman, D.H.: Technicon Monograph No. 3, Geneva, 1968, p. 40.
12. Levy, H.L., and Montag, P.P.: Free amino acids in human amniotic fluid. A quantitative study by ion-exchange chromatography. *Pediatr Res, 3:*113, 1969.
13. Emery, A.E.H., Burt, D., Scrimgeour, J.B., and Nelson, M.M.: Antenatal diagnosis and the amino acid composition of amniotic fluid. *Lancet, 1:*1307, 1970.
14. Morrow, G., III, Schwarz, R.H., Hallock, J.A., and Barness, L.A.: Prenatal detection of methylmalonic acidemia. *J Pediatr, 77:*120, 1970.
15. Seppälä, M., Rouslahti, E., and Tallberg, T.H.: Genetical evidence for maternal origin of amniotic fluid proteins. *Ann Med Exp Biol Fenn, 44:*6, 1966.
16. Dancis, J., Lind, J., and Vera, P.: In Villee, C.A. (Ed.): *The Placental and Foetal Membranes.* Baltimore, Williams & Wilkins, 1960, p. 185.
17. Brzezinski, A., Sadovsky, E., and Shafrir, E.: Electrophoretic distribution of proteins in amniotic fluid and in maternal and fetal serum. *Am J Obstet Gynecol, 82:*800, 1961.
18. Brzezinski, A., Sadovsky, E., and Shafrir, E.: Protein composition of early amniotic fluid and fetal serum with a case of bis-albuminemia. *Am J Obstet Gynecol, 89:*488, 1964.
19. Marks, J.F., Baum, J., Kay, J.L., Taylor, W., and Curry, L.: Amniotic fluid concentrations of uric acid. *Pediatrics, 42:*360, 1968.
20. Baird, C.W., and Bush, I.E.: Cortisone and cortisol contents of amniotic fluid from diabetic and non-diabetic women. *Acta Endocrinol, 34:*97, 1960.
21. Jeffcoate, T.N.A., Fliegner, J.R.H., Russell, S.H., Davis, J.C., and Wade, A.D.: Diagnosis of the adrenogenital syndrome before birth. *Lancet, 2:*553, 1965.

22. Merkatz, I.R., New, M.I., Peterson, R.E., and Seaman, M.P.: Prenatal diagnosis of adrenogenital syndrome by amniocentesis. *J Pediatr, 75:* 977, 1970.
23. Klopper, A.I., and MacNaughton, M.C.: The identification of pregnanediol in liquor amnii, bile and faeces. *J Endocrinol, 18:*319, 1959.
24. Cope, C.L., Hurlock, B., and Swell, C.: The distribution of adrenal cortical hormone in some body fluids. *Clin Sci, 14:*25, 1955.
25. Lambert, M., and Pennington, G.W.: The estimation of polar steroids in liquor amnii. *J Endocrinol, 32:*287, 1965.
26. Abt, K.R., and Keller, M.: 17 Keto-steroids and phenolic steroids in amniotic fluid. *Geburtshilfe Frauenheilkd, 14:*126, 1954.
27. Aleem, F.A., Pinkerton, J.H.M., and Neill, D.W.: Clinical significance of the amniotic fluid oestriol level. *J Obstet Gynaecol Br Commonw, 76:*200, 1969.
28. Diczfalusy, E., and Magnusson, A.M.: Tissue concentration of oestrone, oestradiol, and oestriol in the human fetus. *Acta Endocrinol, 28:*169, 1958.
29. Schindler, A.E., and Herrmann, W.L.: Estriol in pregnancy urine and amniotic fluid. *Am J Obstet Gynecol, 95:*301, 1966.
30. Schindler, A.E., Ratanasopa, V., Lee, T.Y., and Herrmann, W.L.: Estriol and Rh isoimmunization: a new approach to the management of severely affected pregnancies. *Obstet Gynecol, 29:*625, 1967.
31. Troen, P., Nilsson, B., Wiqvist, N., and Diczfalusy, E.: The pattern of estriol conjugates in normal human cord blood, amniotic fluid, and urine of newborns. *Acta Endocrinol, 38:*371, 1961.
32. Bruner, J.A.: Distribution of chorionic gonadotrophin in mother and fetus at various stages of pregnancy. *J Clin Endocrinol, 11:*360, 1951.
33. Tallberg, T., Rouslahti, E., and Ehnholm, C.: Immunological studies on human placental proteins and the purification of the human placental lactogen. *Ann Med Exp Biol Fenn, 43:*67, 1965.
34. Fuchs, F.: Discussion of paper by Jacobson and Barter. *Am J Obstet Gynecol, 99:*806, 1967.
35. Nichols, J.: Antenatal diagnosis and treatment of the adrenogenital syndrome. *Lancet, 1:*83, 1970.
36. Nadler, H.L., and Messina, A.M.: In-utero detection of type-II glycogenosis (Pompe's disease). *Lancet, 2:*1277, 1969.
37. Jung, G., and Diem, R.: Enzyme content of amniotic fluid. *Arch Gynaekol, 192:*155, 1959.
38. McKay, D.G., Richardson, M.V., and Hertig, A.T.: Studies of the function of early human trophoblast. III. A study of the protein structure of mole fluid, chorionic and amniotic fluids by paper electrophoresis. *Am J Obstet Gynecol, 75:*699, 1958.
39. Swelich, F., and Ehrlich-Gomolka, H.: Uber die saure und alkalisch phosphate in placenta und fruchtwasser. *Enzymologia, 15:*96, 1951.

40. Zelnicek, E., and Povarek, J.: Alpha-ketogluteric and pyruvic acids and enzymes in effusions in man. *Clin Chim Acta, 6:*464, 1961.
41. Antonini, E., Fioretti, T., and DeMarco, C.: Glycolytic enzymes in human amniotic fluid. *Experientia, 13:*357, 1957.
42. Von Geyer, H.: Die herkunft der fruchtwasser-Enzyme. *Z Klin Chem Klin Biochem, 8:*145, 1970.
43. Von Geyer, H., and Schneider, I.: Enzyme im fruchtwasser. *Z Klin Chem Klin Biochem, 8:*141, 1970.
44. Toschi, P.: B-glucuronidase activity of serum, amniotic fluid, and cerebral spinal fluid in pre-eclampsia and eclampsia. *Attual Ostet Ginecol, 10:*22, 1964.
45. Bromboszca, A., and Stepniewski, M.: Amniotic fluid and blood serum cholinesterase during labor. *Przegl Lek, 21:*255, 1965.
46. Southren, H.L., Kobayashi, Y., Brenner, T., and Weingold, A.B.: Diamine oxidase activity in the human maternal and fetal plasma and tissues at parturition. *J Appl Physiol, 20:*1048, 1965.
47. Weingold, A.B., and Southren, A.L.: Diamine oxidase as an index of the feto-placental unit. *Obstet Gynecol, 32:*593, 1968.
48. Maeda, K.: Enzymes of the amniotic fluid. *Biochem Z, 144:*1, 1924.
49. Kubli, I.F.: Enzyme studies in amniotic fluid. Lactic dehydrogenase and glutamic-oxalacetic transaminase. *Zentralbl Gynaekol, 83:*1151, 1961.
50. Lin, Y.S.: The components (proteins, phosphatase and transaminase) of human amniotic fluid. *Korean Central J Med, 61:*17, 1964.
51. Uuspaa, V.J.: High histaminase activity of human blood in pregnancy and the so-called placental haemochorialis. *Ann Med Exp Biol Fenn, 29:*81, 1951.
52. Wiegershausen, B., Peagelow, I., Neumayer, E., and Walter, H.: The kininogen content in plasma and amniotic fluid. *Acta Biol Med Ger, 19:*61, 1967.
53. Ckresser, M., and Worashk, H.J.: Determination of leucine aminopeptidase in extracts from the placenta and the placental membranes as well as the amniotic fluid during the early months of pregnancy. *Z Geburtshilfe Gynaekol, 164:*76, 1965.
54. Zsolnai, B., Somogyi, J., Szarvas, Z., and Puskas, E.: The role of proteolytic enzymes in pregnancy. I. The behavior of leucine aminopeptidase in the serum and placenta. *Acta Chir Acad Sci Hung, 5:*207, 1964.
55. Zecchietti, G.: Demonstration of lysozyme in the amniotic fluid, with reference to the bacteriocidal power of the amniotic fluid. *Quad Clin Ostet Ginecol, 3:*233, 1948.
56. Koren, Z.: The significance of mono-amine oxidase in amniotic fluid in human foetal development. *J Obstet Gynaecol Br Commonw, 74:*775, 1967.

57. Brzezinski, A., Koren, Z., Pfeifer, Y., and Sulman, F.G.: The metabolism of serotonin in amniotic fluid. *J Obstet Gynaecol Br Commonw, 69:* 661, 1962.
58. Santoni, G.: Oxidation of p-phenylenediamine by the serum of pregnant women by cord serum and amniotic fluid. Relation to ceruloplasmin content. *Ann Ostet Ginecol, 80:*70, 1958.
59. Nadler, H.L., Bigley, R.H., and Hug, G.: Prenatal detection of Pompe's disease. *Lancet,* in press.
60. Matalon, R., Dorfman, A., Nadler, H., and Jacobson, C.B.: A chemical method for the prenatal diagnosis of mucopolysaccarides. *Lancet, 1:*83, 1970.
61. Van Leeuwen, L., Jacoby, H., and Charles, D.: Exfoliative cytology of amniotic fluid. *Acta Cytol, 9:*442, 1965.
62. Huisjes, H.J.: Origin of the cells in the liquor amnii. *Am J Obstet Gynecol, 106:*1222, 1970.
63. Fuchs, F., and Riis, P.: Antenatal sex determination. *Nature, 177:*330, 1956.
64. Shettles, L.B.: Nuclear morphology of cells in amniotic fluid in relation to sex of infant. *Am J Obstet Gynecol, 71:*834, 1956.
65. Makowski, E.L., Prem, K.A., and Kaiser, I.H.: Detection of sex of fetuses by the incidence of sex chromatin body in nuclei of cells in amniotic fluid. *Science, 123:*542, 1956.
66. Serr, D.M., Sachs, L., and Danon, M.: Diagnosis of sex before birth using cells from amniotic fluid. *Bull Res Council Israel,* 5B137, 1955.
67. Dewhurst, C.J.: Diagnosis of sex before birth. *Lancet, 1:*471, 1956.
68. James, F.: Sexing foetuses by examination of the amniotic fluid. *Lancet, 1:*202, 1956.
69. Keymer, E., Silva-Inzunza, E., and Coutts, W.E.: Contribution to the antenatal determination of sex. *Am J Obstet Gynecol, 74:*1098, 1957.
70. Pasquinucci, C.: Studio della "chromatina sessuale" nelle cellule del liquido amniotico per la diagnosi prenatale di sesso. *Ann Ostet Ginecol, 79:*152, 1957.
71. Amarose, A.P., Wallingford, A.J., and Plotz, E.J.: Prediction of fetal sex from cytologic examination of amniotic fluid. *N Engl J Med, 275:* 715, 1966.
72. Riis, P., and Fuchs, F.: Sex chromatin and antenatal sex diagnosis. In Moore, K.G. (Ed.): *The Sex Chromatin.* Philadelphia, Saunders, 1966.
73. Serr, D.M., and Margolis, E.: Diagnosis of fetal sex in a sex-linked hereditary disorder. *Am J Obstet Gynecol, 88:*230, 1964.
74. Nadler, H.L., and Gerbie, A.B.: Role of amniocentesis in the intrauterine detection of genetic disorders. *N Engl J Med, 282:*596, 1970.
75. Fuchs, F., Freiesleben, E., Knudsen, E.E., and Riis, P.: Determination of foetal blood-group. *Lancet, 1:*996, 1956.

76. Sachs, L., Feldman, M., and Danon, M.: Prenatal identification of blood group antigens. *Lancet, 2:*356, 1956.
77. Broussy, J., Ducos, J., and Baux, R.: Mise en evidence des antigenes A et B dans le liquide amniotique humain et en. *C R Soc Biol, 152:*172, 1958.
78. Gordon, H., and Brosens, I.: Cytology of amniotic fluid: a new test for fetal maturity. *Obstet Gynecol, 30:*652, 1967.
79. Hug, G., Schubert, W.K., and Soukup, S.: Prenatal diagnosis of type-II glycogenosis. *Lancet, 1:*1002, 1970.
80. Cox, R.P., Douglas, G., Hutzler, J., Lynfield, J., and Dancis, J.: In-utero detection of Pompe's disease. *Lancet, 1:*893, 1970.
81. Kaback, M.M.: Personal communication.
82. Berman, P.H., Balis, M.E., and Dancis, J.: A method for the prenatal diagnosis of congenital hyperuricemia. *J Pediatr, 75:*488, 1969.
83. Nadler, H.L., and Gerbie, A.B.: Enzymes in noncultured amniotic fluid cells. *Am J Obstet Gynecol, 103:*710, 1969.
84. Sutcliffe, R.G., and Brock, D.J.H.: Enzymes in uncultured amniotic fluid cells. Personal communication.
85. O'Brien, J.S.: Lipid Storage Disease. Conference on Antenatal Detection of Genetic Disorders. Chicago, June, 1970.
86. Rattazzi, M.C., and Davidson, R.G.: Prenatal Detection of Tay-Sachs Disease. Presented at the Meeting on Antenatal Diagnosis. Chicago, June 11-12, 1970.
87. Dancis, J.: The antepartum diagnosis of genetic diseases. *J Pediatr, 72:*301, 1968.
88. Schneck, L., Valenti, C., Amsterdam, D., Friedland, J., Adachi, M., and Volk, B.W.: Prenatal diagnosis of Tay-Sachs disease. *Lancet, 1:*582, 1970.
89. Jacobson, C.B., and Barter, R.H. Intra-uterine diagnosis and management of genetic defects. *Am J Obstet Gynecol, 99:*796, 1967.
90. Steele, M.W., and Breg, W.R.: Chromosome analysis of human amniotic fluid cells. *Lancet, 1:*383, 1966.
91. Thiede, H.A., Creasman, W.T., and Metcalfe, S.: Antenatal analysis of the human chromosomes. *Am J Obstet Gynecol 94:*589, 1966.
92. Emery, A.E. (Ed.): *Modern Trends in Human Genetics.* Great Britain, Butterworths, 1970, p. 267.
93. Uhlendorf, B.W., Jacobson, C.B., Sloan, H.R., Mudd, S.H., Herndon, J.H., Brady, R.O., Seegmiller, J.E., and Fujimoto, W.: Cell Cultures Derived from Human Amniotic Fuid: Their Possible Application in the Intra-uterine Diagnosis of Heritable Metabolic Disease. Nineteenth Annual Meeting of the Tissue Culture Association, Schedule and Abstracts, San Juan, 1968, *In Vitro,* p. 158.
94. Lisgar, F., Gertner, M., Cherry, S., Hsu, L.Y., and Hirschhorn, K.: Prenatal chromosome analysis. *Nature, 225:*280, 1970.

95. Abbo, G., and Zellweger, H.: Prenatal determination of fetal sex and chromosomal complement. *Lancet, 1:*216, 1970.
96. Gregson, N.M.: A technique for culturing cells from amniotic fluid. *Lancet, 1:*84, 1970.
97. Santesson, B., Akesson, H.-O., Böök, J.A., and Brosset, A.: Karyotyping human amniotic fluid cells. *Lancet, 2:*1067, 1969.
98. Valenti, C., and Kehaty, T.: Culture of cells obtained by amniocentesis. *J Lab Clin Med, 73:*355, 1969.
99. Nelson, M.M., and Emery, A.E.H.: Amniotic fluid cells; prenatal sex prediction and culture. *Br Med J, 1:*523, 1970.
100. Nadler, H.L., Gerbie, A., Jacobson, C.B., Valenti, C., and Macintyre, M.N.: In preparation.
101. Gerbie, A.B., and Nadler, H.L.: Amniocentesis in genetic counseling. *Am J Obstet Gynecol,* in press.
102. Valenti, C., Schutta, E.J., and Kehaty, T.: Prenatal diagnosis of Down's syndrome. *Lancet, 2:*220, 1968.
103. Gertner, M., Hsu, L.Y., and Hirschhorn, K.: The use of amniocentesis in genetic counseling. *Proc Soc Pediatr Res,* Atlantic City, May 2, 1970, p. 125.
104. Uhlendorf, B.W.: Personal communication.
105. Nadler, H.L.: Patterns of enzyme development using cultivated human fetal cells from amniotic fluid. *Biochem Genet 2:*119, 1968.
106. Nadler, H.L.: Unpublished data.
107. Shih, V.E., Littlefield, J.W., and Moser, H.W.: Personal communication.
108. Sloan, H.R., Uhlendorf, B.W., Jacobson, C.B., and Fredrickson, D.S.: β-galactosidase in tissue culture derived from human skin and bone marrow: enzyme defect in G_{M1} gangliosidosis. *Pediatr Res, 3:*532, 1969.
109. Beutler, E., Kuhl, W., Trinidad, F., Teplitz, R., and Nadler, H.: β-glucosidase activity in fibroblasts from homozygotes and heterozygotes from Gaucher's disease. *Lancet,* in press.
110. Uhlendorf, B.W., and Mudd, S.H.: Cystathionine synthase in tissue culture derived from human skin: Enzyme defect in homocystinuria. *Science, 160:*1007, 1968.
111. Okada, S., and O'Brien, J.S.: Tay-Sachs disease: generalized absence of a Beta-D-N-acetylhexosaminidase component. *Science, 165:*698, 1969.
112. Fujimoto, W.Y., Seegmiller, J.E., Uhlendorf, B.W., and Jacobson, C.B.: Biochemical diagnosis of an X-linked disease *in utero. Lancet, 2:*511, 1968.
113. DeMars, R., Sarto, G., Felix, J.S., and Benke, P.: Lesch-Nyhan mutation: prenatal detection with amniotic fluid cells. *Science, 164:*1303, 1969.

114. Kaback, M.M., Leonard, C.O., and Parmley, T.H.: Intra-uterine diagnosis: comparative enzymology of fibroblasts cultivated from maternal skin, fetal skin, and amniotic fluid cells. *Proc Soc Pediatr Res,* Atlantic City, May 2, 1970, p. 27.

115. Nadler, H.L.: Antenatal detection of hereditary disorders. *Pediatrics, 42:*912, 1968.

116. Fratantoni, J.C., Neufeld, E.F., Uhlendorf, B.W., and Jacobson, C.B.: Intra-uterine diagnosis of the Hurler and Hunter syndromes. *N Engl J Med, 280:*686, 1969.

117. Nadler, H.L., Wodnicki, J.M., Swae, M.A., and O'Flynn, M.E.: Cultivated amniotic fluid cells and fibroblasts derived from families with cystic fibrosis. *Lanet, 2:*84, 1969.

118. Nadler, H.L., and Egan, T.J.: Deficiency of lysosomal acid phosphatase: A new familial metabolic disorder. *N Engl J Med, 282:*302, 1970.

119. Valenti, C., Schutta, E.J., and Kehaty, T.: Cytogenetic diagnosis of Down's syndrome *in utero. JAMA, 207:*1513, 1969.

120. Justice, P., Ryan, C., and Hsia, D.Y.Y.: Amylo-1,6-glucosidase in human fibroblasts: Studies in type III glycogen storage disease. *Biochem Biophys Res Commun, 39:*301, 1970.

121. Schulman, J.D., Fujimoto, W.Y., Bradley, K.H., and Seegmiller, J.E.: Identification of the heterozygous genotype for cystinosis *in utero.* Personal communication.

122. Andrews, B.F.: Amniotic fluid studies to determine maturity. *Pediatr Clin North Am, 17:*49, 1970.

123. Mandelbaum, B., La Croix, G.C., and Robinson, A.R.: Determination of fetal maturity by spectrophotometric analysis of amniotic fluid. *Obstet Gynecol, 29:*471, 1967.

124. Cherry, S.H.: Amniotic fluid bilirubin as an index of fetal maturity. *Obstet Gynecol, 30:*615, 1967.

125. White, C.A., Doorenbos, D.E., and Bradbury, J.T.: Role of chemical and cytological analysis of amniotic fluid in determination of fetal maturity. *Am J Obstet Gynecol, 104:*664, 1969.

126. Wiser, W.L., and Thiede, H.A.: Amniotic fluid and fetal maturity. *South Med J, 62:*755, 1969.

127. Liley, A.W.: Liquor amnii analysis in the management of the pregnancy complicated by rhesus sensitization. *Am J Obstet Gynecol, 82:*1359, 1961.

128. Woyton, J.: Assessment of fetal maturity based on examination of liquor amnii. *J Zbl Gynak, 85:*552, 1963. (Abstracted, *J Obstet Gynaecol Br Commonw, 70:*907, 1963.)

129. Begneaud, W.P., Hawes, T.P., Mickal, A., and Samuels, M.: Amniotic fluid creatinine for prediction of fetal maturity. *Obstet Gynecol, 34:*7, 1969.

130. Pitkin, R.M., and Zwirek, S.J.: Amniotic fluid creatinine. *Am J Obstet Gynecol, 98:*1135, 1967.
131. Miles, P.A., and Pearson, J.W.: Amniotic fluid osmolality in assessing fetal maturity. *Obstet Gynecol, 34:*701, 1969.
132. Seeds, A.E., Jr.: Amniotic fluid and fetal water metabolism. In Barnes, A.C. (Ed.): *Intra-uterine Development.* Philadelphia, Lea & Febiger, 1968, p. 129.
133. Kittrich, M.: Cytodiagnosis of amniotic fluid discharge by means of nile blue. *Geburtshilfe Frauenheilkd, 23:*156, 1963.
134. Brosens, I.A.: Cytological study of amniotic fluid with nile blue sulfate staining. *Acta Cytol, 10:*159, 1966.
135. Brosens, I.A., and Gordon, H.: An estimation of maturity by cytological examination of the liquor amnii. *J Obstet Gynaecol Br Commonw, 73:*88, 1966.
136. Brosens, I.A., and Gordon, H.: Cytology of amniotic fluid. *Obstet Gynecol, 30:*652, 1967.
137. Bishop, E.H., and Corson, S.: Estimation of fetal maturity by cytological examination of amniotic fluid. *J Obstet Gynecol, 102:*654, 1968.
138. Graven, S.N.: Phospholipids in human and monkey amniotic fluid. *Proc Soc Pediatr Res,* 1968, p. 52.
139. Nelson, G.H.: Amniotic fluid phospholipid patterns in normal and abnormal pregnancies. *Am J Obstet Gynecol, 105:*1072, 1969.
140. Gluck, L., Kulovich, M.V., Borer, R.C., Jr., Brenner, P.H., Anderson, G.G., and Spellacy, W.N.: The Biochemical Development of Surface Activity in Mammalian Lung: V. Maturity of the Fetal Lung; Predicting Fetal Outcome with Respect to the Respiratory Distress Syndrome (RDS) by Amniotic Fluid Phospholipids. In preparation.
141. Scarpelli, E.M.: The lung, tracheal fluid, and lipid metabolism of the fetus. *Pediatrics, 40:*951, 1967.

Chapter 6

AMNIOTIC FLUID IN THE RH-SENSITIZED PATIENT

BRIAN LITTLE

From the time that the Rh factor was demonstrated to be the cause of hemolytic anemia in the newborn[60] there has been a general dissatisfaction with the ability either to predict the presence of an Rh-negative fetus when the anti-Rh titer was high or to anticipate intrauterine fetal death with maternal antibody titer alone.[23] More recent studies have proposed the administration of anti-Rh antibody postpartum to Rh-negative mothers with Rh-positive infants, which will reduce to negligible proportions the incidence of sensitized women in subsequent pregnancies. However, amniocentesis with examination of amniotic fluid has been a singular contribution to the evaluation of the fetus *in utero.* It has taken nearly 20 years since the earliest observations of Bevis[15] for the method of amniocentesis and amniotic fluid evaluation to become adopted and accepted as an integral part of the care of the Rh-sensitized mother.

INDICATIONS FOR AMNIOCENTESIS

The indications that many investigators give for amniocentesis in sensitized Rh-negative pregnant women are somewhat different. However, investigators all agree that the woman must have a positive Rh antibody titer before amniotic fluid is drawn for evalution. There has been varying agreement as to the value of an Rh antibody titer in anticipating the prognosis for the fetus. Saline titers (measuring complete antibodies, IgM, 19S) were replaced by albumin titers and the Coombs' titer (measuring incomplete antibodies, IgG, 7S). Some laboratories took great pains to establish levels of titer and the reproducibility of their methods, but at best it was an imprecise measurement of the state of the fetus *in utero,* for results could only be standardized to ± one dilution.

Most recently quantitative hemagglutinin assays have been established using bromelin and polyvinylpyrrolidone. Quantitative assays of the nitrogen content of gamma G globulin per milliliter of serum have been measured which make titers much more exact. No treatment was required for the Rh-positive babies at values below 0.1 μg of nitrogen per milliliter of serum in sensitized mothers.[99, 100]

Most laboratories now use titers of 1:8, 1:16 or 1:64 (albumin titer) as an indication for amniocentesis in a previously unaffected mother. The initial amniocentesis on a previously unaffected patient is usually carried out between 28 and 32 weeks' gestation. Walker[110] has given some guidelines for patients who require management for rhesus iso-immunization:

1. Previous infant Coombs' positive but no treatment required (10% of all cases): In these cases the risk of stillbirth is small; therefore, spontaneous delivery is planned unless there is a clinical indication for further tests.

2. Previous infant stillborn or very severely affected (10% of all cases): Liquor examination is carried out from 20 weeks' gestation onwards.

3. Previous infant Coombs' positive and treatment required (20% of all cases): Amniocentesis is carried out at 32 weeks' gestation and, if necessary, repeated at 35 weeks' gestation.

4. First affected cases (60% of all cases): Amniocentesis is carried out at 32 weeks' gestation and, if necessary, at 35 weeks' gestation provided that the antibody titer is 1:16 or higher.

Bowman and Pollock[24] describe the indications for amniocentesis in Winnipeg, Canada, which are remarkably similar to Walker's general guidelines:

1. In all iso-immunized cases with a history of preceding disease causing stillbirth, or severe enough to require treatment.

2. In all iso-immunized pregnancies with a preceding history of stillbirth, cause unknown.

3. In all first sensitized cases in which antibody titer exceeds 8 in albumin by the 32nd week of gestation.

4. In all second and subsequent sensitized pregnancies in which

the previous baby did not require treatment and the titer is 16 in albumin or higher.

Walker's conservative approach is based on the outcome of previous pregnancies. However, many clinics now believe that amniocentesis is a relatively benign procedure; these clinics carry out the first antibody tests earlier and do amniocentesis when the titer is 1:8. Amniocentesis in the most severe cases has been done as early as 16 weeks' gestation in anticipation of a possible intrauterine transfusion. This early invasion of the amniotic cavity is becoming more common as investigation and identification of abnormal fetal karyotypes from amniotic fluid cultures is being done. The decision to do amniocentesis should be made with care and should be based on both past history and maternal titer, as the procedure does carry a small but real risk of complications.[111]

AMNIOCENTESIS

The procedure of amniocentesis is now well known. The use of a sharp #22 disposable spinal needle is most common. Whereas some like to admit patients to the hospital for the amniocentesis, this is not generally done. There is little danger of serious complication provided that the bladder is empty, that there are no adhesions from previous operations, and that the needle is aimed away from the vital areas of the fetus and placenta. There have been reports of premature labor, infection, and damage to the fetus, particularly when a chorionic vessel has been damaged. Fetal death has been reported, but this is rare.[54] It must be remembered that in the Rh-negative woman who has an Rh-positive child *in utero* there is the possibility of sensitization and further immunization from the procedure itself. Increased titers (anti-D) in mothers' blood and the presence of fetal red blood cells in the maternal circulation have been demonstrated following amniocentesis,[93] but there appears to be no proof that the severity of the disease is affected.[37]

The amniotic fluid should be protected from direct light and sunlight, for bilirubin decomposes by photo-oxidation in light. Protection from heat and freezing are not quite so important. Some investigators actually freeze the fluid for storage, and heating has to be greater than 60° C before there is more than 15 percent loss of bilirubin in the amniotic fluid.[77] Amniotic fluid should be filtered or centrifuged (millipore filters do not appear to have any advantage over filter paper)[34] and examined as soon as possible after being drawn to eliminate as many methodological errors as feasible.

AMNIOTIC FLUID EVALUATION HISTORY

In the September 1950 *Lancet,* D.C.A. Bevis, then Senior Registrar at St. Mary's Hospital, Manchester, addressed himself to the "composition of the liquor amnii in haemolytic disease of the newborn." He reported that "attempts to demonstrate the presence of bile-pigments with Fouchet's reagent and the van den Bergh reaction proved negative in all cases, including two in which the liquor had the characteristic golden colour seen in severe haemolytic disease."

Ironically enough, responding to Bevis' original preliminary communication in a letter addressed to the editor of the *Lancet,* Gairdner, Lawrie and Hutcheon[45] of the Cambridge Maternity Hospital, Cambridge, described six cases in which "it appears that coloured bilirubin-containing liquor tends to be associated with severe forms of the disease. However, coloured liquor is sometimes found in normals." Examining "normal" amniotic fluid they found six fluids (59 subjects) were colored green or yellow. In three there was a concentration of bilirubin of 0.5 to 1.2 mg/100 ml, but three failed to react to the van den Bergh reagents. They demonstrated that meconium could not only account for the greenish color, but also that a 1.25% suspension of meconium had a bilirubin content of 1.6 mg/100 ml. They believed that the bilirubin they saw in the sensitized women's amniotic fluid might come from the presence of meconium. In conclusion, they stated that "the bilirubin content of liquor might provide some guide to the degree of involvement of the fetus by haemolytic disease. But from Mr. Bevis' work it seems that the iron content is more likely to prove of use in this sense."

Bevis, however, proposed that "the concentration of non-haematin iron and urobilinogen in liquor amnii offer a reliable guide to the outcome of the foetus."[14] The estimation of nonhematin iron was plotted in a semilogarithmic plot against the hemoglobin concentration of cord blood. The hematologic status of the fetus could be anticipated by the amniotic fluid nonhematin iron concentration. In addition, if the concentration of urobilinogen in the amniotic fluid was observed to fall, the prognosis was grave. Later Bevis examined the icterus index of the amniotic fluid, compared it with bilirubin content, and pointed out the discrepancy between the two and the difficulty of prognosis for babies with respect to the development of kernicterus.[16] In 1956, the first spectral curves were carried out on amniotic fluid by Bevis,[17] and the elucidation of various pigments in both liquor amnii and cord blood was used as an indication of the severity of the hemolytic process in the baby. Bilirubin, oxyhemoglobin, methemalbumin, and vernix were examined as individual pigments absorbing light and contributing to the final spectral curve obtained from amniotic fluid in the sensitized mother. At that time, there was strong resistance to the premature delivery of sensitized infants.[17] Armitage and Mollison[9] and Allen[8] were strongly urging that premature delivery not be used as a routine procedure in the management of the Rh-sensitized mother. Although Bevis did not propose delivery as early as it was subsequently carried out, he did suggest that some babies were seriously affected in the last few weeks by the sudden onset of severe hemolytic process and that the assessment of the fetus by amniotic fluid examination and delivery with immediate replacement transfusion had a definite place in selected cases. In an attempt to obtain quantitative results from the spectrophotometric curves, Bevis pointed out that absorption curves of oxyhemoglobin, methemalbumin and protein (which he presumed to be vernix) all followed Beer's law, but that bilirubin did not. This made it necessary to construct curves for bilirubin at different concentrations in amniotic fluid in order to be able to interpret the unknown specimens. Amniotic fluid contains reduced concentration of protein with increasing gestational age and, with the development of erythroblastosis in the fetus, the protein concentration does not fall and in severe cases actually increases.

Freda and Gorman[41] used a recording spectrophotometer to demonstrate curves for normal amniotic fluid. Linear graphs of optical density showed decreased absorption with increased wavelength. "Humps" occurred in the curve at 450 mμ in the presence of hemolytic disease of the fetus. No effort was made in these studies to quantitate the "humps" or correct for background, and only general conclusions were stated.

Although Bevis[17] described a composite curve with a peak at 460 mμ, A. H. C. Walker[108] described the fact that the optical density at various wavelengths was a straight line from 600 to 400 mμ in unaffected cases but that there was a "bulge" at 450 mμ when the baby was affected by hemolytic disease. Walker described the first 101 cases examined in Manchester. When the severity of the disease and the concentration of bilirubin considered as the "height of the bulge" were correlated, an accurate prediction was obtained in 95 percent of the cases tested early. He observed that amniotic fluid must be tested fresh before 35 weeks and that, paradoxically, in later pregnancy the severity of the disease may be masked by a higher background and turbidity which obliterated the "bulge" (Fig. 6-1).

Cary[29] in Sydney and Mackay[71] in Melbourne, Australia, were actively carrying out amniotic fluid evaluation by 1960. Cary reported 40 cases, but his observations were, at most, only evaluations of the peak at 450 mμ by eye, although his results were encouraging. E. V. Mackay,[71] basing prognosis on the shape of the spectrophotometric curves (which were graded 0 to 5, according to the extent of staining in the fluid), obtained satisfactory results in determining the severity of hemolytic disease in the fetus. Similar observations and curve classifications were adopted independently by Mayer et al.[76] Mackay and Watson[72] then correlated their spectrophotometric observations with direct chemical bilirubin estimations using Watson's[115] modification of Lathe and Ruthven's[61] diazo method. Exchange transfusion was only rarely necessary when the liquor concentration of bilirubin was below 0.12 mg/100 ml. Their normal values in the presence of Rh-negative infants were range 0-0.11, mean 0.05 mg/100 ml; whereas Bevis stated the mean to be 0.16 ± 0.13 mg/100 ml using a spec-

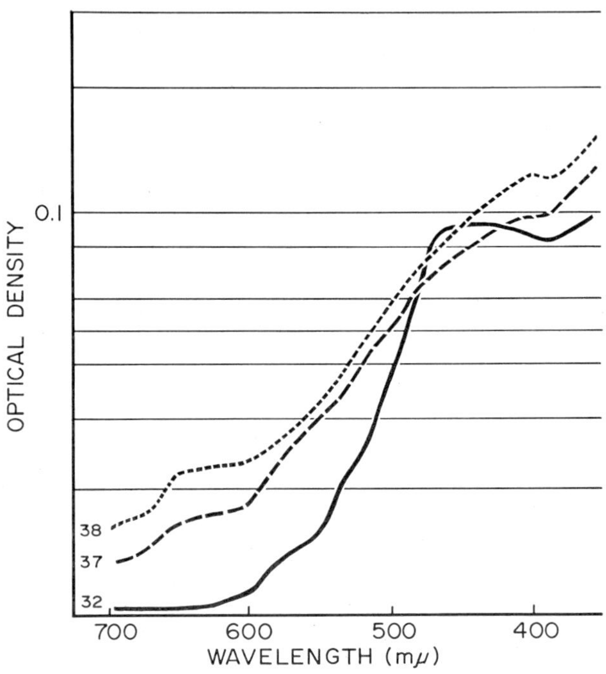

FIGURE 6-1. Three spectrophotometric absorption curves at 32, 37 and 38 weeks in the same patient. All specimens of amniotic fluid were pale and clear. Note the obliteration of the "bulge" with increasing gestation. (From Walker, A. H. C.[108])

trophotometric method with multiple concentrations as standards. As bilirubin does not follow Beer's law, other investigators showed varying values (see Table 6-I). Mackay and Watson also presented a practical scheme of management of sensitized patients for the induction of labor at various gestational ages based on the liquor bilirubin concentration.

QUANTITATIVE EVALUATION OF SPECTROPHOTOMETRIC CURVES OBTAINED FROM AMNIOTIC FLUID

Liley[64] borrowed from Bevis[15] and A. H. C. Walker[108] and improved on their data to present more quantitative data on the severity of the expected anemia in the prognosis for the fetus as related to the peak of amniotic fluid at 450 mμ. Liley's mea-

TABLE 6-I

BILIRUBIN IN NORMAL AMNIOTIC FLUID DETERMINED BY BIOCHEMICAL METHODS

Author	*Year*	*Bilirubin mg/100 ml*	*Weeks of Gestation*
Bevis[17]	1956	0, 16 ± 0, 13	
Black[20]	1969	≤ 0, 4	28 - 32
Broderson[27]	1968	0, 02	
Fikentscher[40]	1969	0, 03 — 0, 06	
Mast[75]	1969	0, 026 — 0, 094	27 - 41
Morris[83]	1967	0, 05 — 0, 14	30 - 32
Stewart[106]	1967	0, 035 — 0, 060	≥ 38
A. H. C. Walker[109]	1962	≤ 0, 09	≥ 38
A. H. C. Walker[109]	1962	≤ 0, 31	≥ 35
Watson[116]	1965	0, 04	32 - 33
Wild[119]	1961	0, 24	< 35
Wild[119]	1961	0, 10	> 35

from Bartsch[5a]

surement of the optical density at the 450 mμ peak, which he used for prognosis, was actually the difference between the peak and a tangential straight line drawn to the curve plotted in a semi-logarithmic plot (log of OD vs. wavelength) and was later described as ΔOD_{450} (Fig. 6-2). He made several important observations about the amniotic fluid:

1. At 28 to 33 weeks' gestation normal amniotic fluid frequently showed a conspicuous bulge at 450 mμ in affected cases.

2. Pigment peaks had a half-life of 10 hours in laboratory daylight and 12 to 18 minutes in strong sunlight, and, therefore, fluids must be protected from light.

3. Fetal blood could contaminate the sample, as fetal serum was known to have a higher concentration of the pigments measured than the amniotic fluid, and care should be taken to observe such contamination.

4. Patients with a history of antepartum hemorrhage could have either free maternal hemoglobin (A) in the amniotic fluid

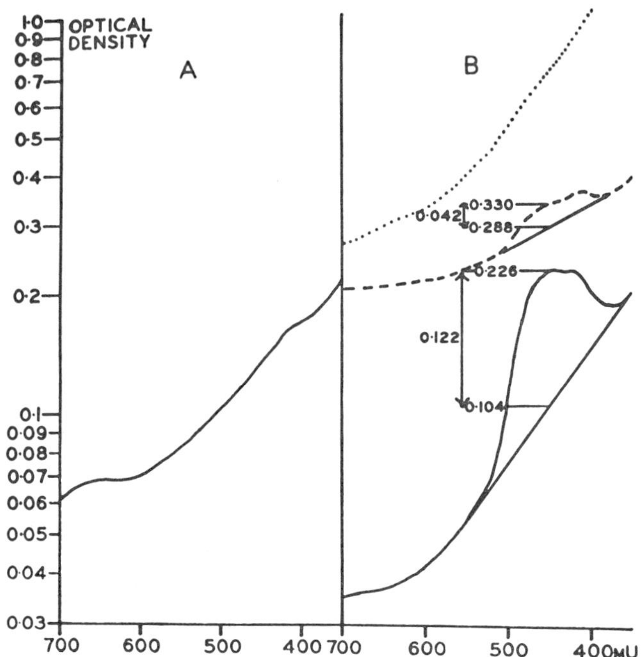

FIGURE 6-2. A, "Negative curve." A spectral absorption curve from an Rh-sensitized woman with an unaffected baby. B, "Positive curve." Absorption curves of amniotic fluid at 31 weeks (solid line), 35½ weeks (dashed line) and 38 weeks (dotted line) from a pregnancy resulting in an affected baby with a cord hemoglobin of 13 gm/100 ml at 38 weeks. Note the method of calculating the 450 mμ peak (Δ OD_{450}). (From Liley.[64])

or absorb enough bilirubin from the site of the hemorrhage be it retroplacental, retrochorionic, or fetal to affect the spectrophotometric reading at 450 mμ.

5. Oxyhemoglobin contamination, usually an artefact, could be corrected for by subtracting 5 percent of the peak at 415 mμ from the 450 mμ peak.

6. He confirmed A. H. C. Walker's [108] observation that some peaks of absorption at 450 mμ may diminish with increasing maturity of the fetus.

Liley[64] then presented the data from 101 cases and indicated that "the severity of the hemolytic disease could be predicted by considering the size and trend of the 450 mμ peak in liquor in relation to 3 zones" (now usually referred to as Liley Zones I, II and III) (Fig. 6-3). He also demonstrated an indirect association between the optical density (OD) peak at 450 mμ and the cord hemoglobin when delivery occurred within one week ($r = 0.87$), whereas correlation between OD_{450} peak and cord bilirubin or cord bilirubin and cord hemoglobin was not as good ($r = +0.29$ and $r = -0.38$) although the latter correlation was significant ($p < .01$). The occasional (9 out of 101) aspiration of fetal blood indicated caution in interpretation of large pigment peaks, but was helpful in determining fetal blood type for transfusion and confirming any conflict between the amniotic fluid reading and the behavior of the antibody titer and past history. While confirming Bevis' observation of high nonhematin iron ($> 40 \mu g/100$ ml) as indicating severe anemia in the fetus, he showed that even when values were less than $40 \mu g/100$ ml the fetus could be severely afflicted. Liley concluded that such iron estimations did not provide as much guidance as the peaks of absorption at 450 mμ. Liley also indicated that the biochemical estimation of bilirubin seemed an unnecessary refinement and possible complications could ensue because of some of the errors inherent in interpretation of the amniotic fluid values from other contaminants. Liley[65] subsequently elicited "the pitfalls, errors and limits of accuracy in the antenatal prediction of the severity of hemolytic disease from amniotic fluid." Sources of error were in obtaining the wrong fluid, measuring the wrong pigment or obtaining pigment (bilirubin) from a wrong source (e.g. fetal serum) and making a wrong prediction. Maternal urine, fetal ascitic fluid, multiple amniotic sacs, and amniotic cysts can provide samples of wrong fluid. Serum, hemoglobin, meconium, and regurgitation from a fetus with duodenal atresia contributed wrong pigment. Wrong dates and altered maturity at delivery from those assumptions on which predictions had been made accounted for wrong prediction. From these data Liley constructed his well-known graph of the percentage probability of the various grades of affliction of the fetus for the peak size in a single specimen (Fig. 6-4).

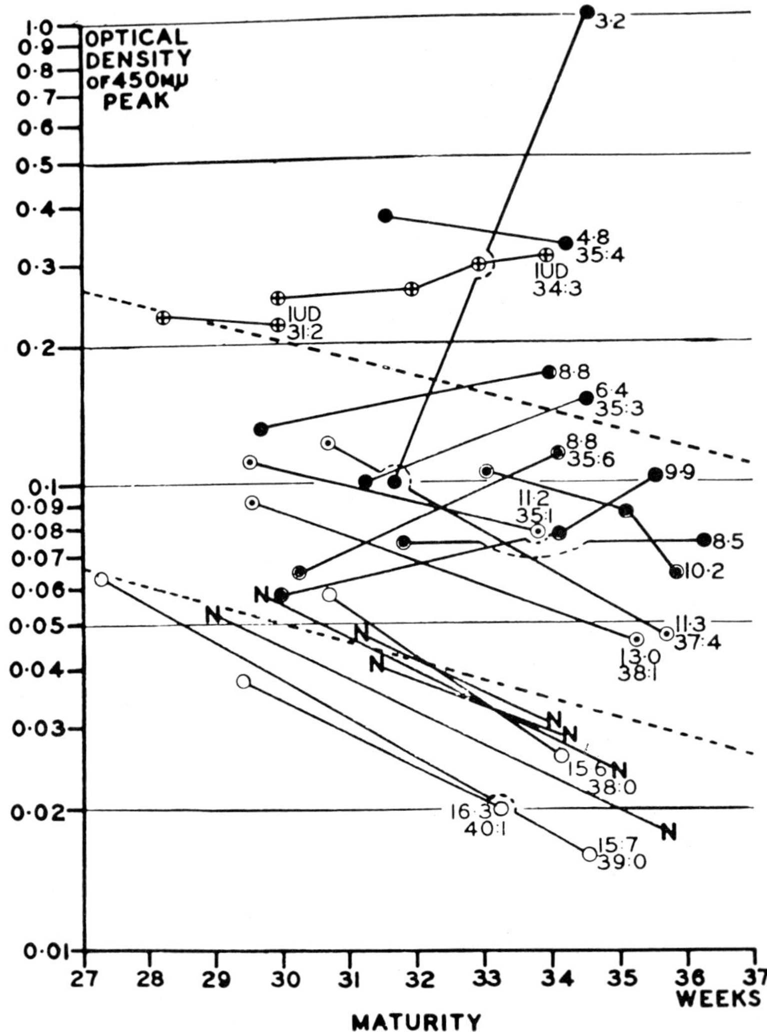

FIGURE 6-3. Examples of the behavior of the 450 mμ peak in 20 pregnancies and the clinical results. The upper figure of each pair indicates cord hemoglobin in grams per 100 ml; the lower figure, maturity at delivery in weeks and days (omitted where the hemoglobin value is simultaneous with the pigment peak). With intrauterine death, the maturity at that event is recorded.

Key		*Hemoglobin gm/100 ml*
○	=	14 or more
⊙	=	11 - 13.9
•	=	8 - 10.9
⊕	=	7.9 or less
+	=	Intrauterine death
N	=	Unaffected

Note the two dashed lines. The lowest is Zone I, the middle Zone II, and the upper Zone III. (From Liley.[64])

Walker, Fairweather and Jones[113] at the University of Newcastle upon Tyne studied 277 liquor specimens from 277 immunized Rh-negative women. They gave a value for "estimated" bilirubin in units, which was the percentage difference between the observed curve and one drawn arbitrarily to omit the bilirubin band. They plotted their values in a semilogarithmic plot of percent transmittance against wavelength from data obtained on an Optica double beam recording spectrophotometer using an 0.5 cm light path and distilled water as blank. Liley[64] had used a Unicam SP 500 or SP 600 and glass or silica cuvettes with a 1.0 cm light path. This difference can cause considerable confusion in comparison of results. Nelson and Talledo[85] resolved this problem somewhat by the recent study of different spectrophotometers. They found that most spectrophotometers will read similar results for a sample of amniotic fluid except the Coleman Junior. This spectrophotometer's wavelength does not extend below 400 mμ, whereas optical density readings must be obtained through 350 mμ in order to achieve a complete curve. However, the length of light path is obviously of importance; a ΔOD_{450} of 0.29 in a 10 mm cell will read as high as 0.46 in a 17 mm cuvette. Care must also be exercised in knowing whether the spectrophotometer records linear OD vs. logarithmic wavelength, linear OD vs. linear wavelength or logarithmic OD vs. linear wavelength, for this can lead to as much as a 30 percent difference in ΔOD_{450} results (Fig. 6-5).

Walker et al.[113] made an effort to be accurate and determined a "calculated" bilirubin which was the optical density at 450 mμ minus the optical density at 412 mμ. This gave the same results

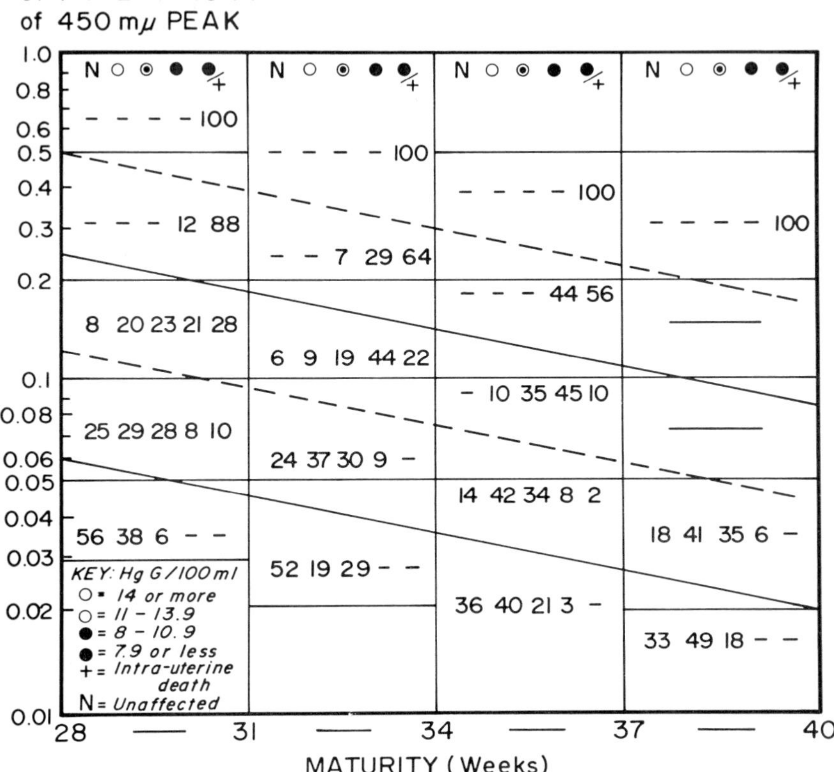

FIGURE 6-4. Percentage probability of the various grades of affliction for the peak size in a single specimen. The solid lines divide the graph into Liley Zones I, II and III from the bottom, up. (From Liley.[65])

as the method of subtracting OD_{575} from OD_{450} ($OD_{450} - OD_{575}$) proposed by White, Haidar and Reinhold[117] for estimating bilirubin in cord blood serum of affected newborn infants. This calculation was made to correct for the contribution of hemoglobin to the light absorption at 450 mμ. The comparison between "estimated," "calculated," and chemically estimated bilirubin was made (the latter by the method of King and Coxon) and an imprecise relationship was found. It was concluded that "estimated" bilirubin in units (which for practical purposes is the same as Liley's OD difference) gave the best correlation with the severity of the

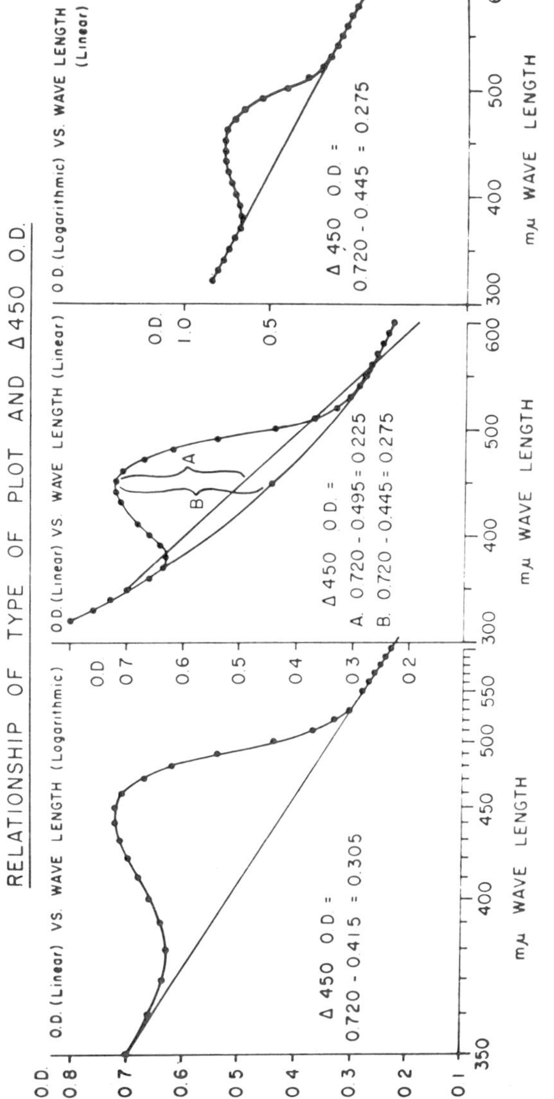

FIGURE 6-5. Spectrum of amniotic fluid from a sensitized pregnancy with Δ OD_{450} calculated from various types of plots. (From Nelson and Talledo.[85])

disease in the fetus. In their observations of protein concentration in amniotic fluid, high protein concentrations were generally associated with high bilirubin concentration. Although the best discrimination among cases was found at liquor protein concentrations greater than 200 mg/100 ml, protein concentration was not as good as "estimated" bilirubin to anticipate the severity of disease in the fetus. Their conclusions, made before the advent of possible intrauterine transfusion, were conservative. Anticipating a forecast of severe disease or stillbirth in at best 50 percent of the cases, they believed amniotic fluid examination would be of special value for those in whom premature induction was being considered or in families where the father was heterozygous and the anamnestic response of the Rh antibody titer proved confusing in establishing the state of the fetus.

While many clinics were debating the value of amniocentesis and spectrophotometric examination of the amniotic fluid in the decision for the early induction of labor, Liley[66] at the National Women's Hospital in Auckland, New Zealand, had been demonstrating its value. With selective induction based on the findings from amniocentesis their perinatal mortality in Rh-sensitized pregnancies dropped from 22 percent in 1957-58 to 9 percent in 1962. When, in 80 cases, there were seven perinatal deaths of which six were hydropic before 34 weeks' gestation, Liley considered intrauterine transfusion as a "logical procedure for these very severely affected babies early in the third trimester." Although his first three attempts ended in failure, his fourth was successful and introduced an era of hope for Rh-sensitized patients who up to then had had an impossible prognosis. The concept of depositing blood cells in the peritoneal cavity of the fetus was novel for younger obstetricians, although their older pediatric colleagues, when pressed for memories, could think back to the time when anemic infants were transfused with blood intraperitoneally.[79] The blood is apparently absorbed through lymphatics in the diaphragm and deposited by way of the thoracic duct and similar channels into the vena cava. This possibility, therefore, puts a much greater burden on the evaluation of amniotic fluid; for the decision to carry out an intrauterine transfusion, rather than an early induction of labor, carries with it the possibility of considerable morbidity and mortality of both fetus and mother.

AMNIOTIC FLUID CONTENT

With an increasing interest in and availability of amniotic fluid, more and more tests are being carried out at all stages of gestation to determine possible correlations with the state of the fetus. Liquor protein concentration, electrolyte composition, chorionic gonadotrophin content, estriol content and creatinine concentration are all being measured as indications of the state of the fetus. The fluid from sensitized women is also being examined chemically as well as spectrophotometrically. Whereas Liley's previously quoted comment that additional estimations on the amniotic fluid in addition to the spectrophotometric evaluation appeared to be an "unnecessary refinement" for the management of such pregnancies, he would be the last to suggest that such measurements would not give us additional leads which would be of help in some of the problems which have, and may still, develop in such management.

PROTEIN CONCENTRATION

Although early reports by Mentasti[80] and Abbas and Tovey[7] report an increase in concentration of protein in the amniotic fluid of four cases of hemolytic disease (in two of which cases hydropic infants were delivered), Wild[119] has taken one of the first definitive looks at the association between protein and bilirubin in amniotic fluid. Wild's interest apparently grew out of his association with Walker and Jennison in Manchester.

The amniotic fluids of 72 mothers were examined for protein concentration by a method of Kingsbury, Clark, Williams and Post (described in a text by Varley[4]) comparing amniotic fluid with standards of serum proteins between 0 and 100 mg/100 ml at 660 mμ. The bilirubin was estimated by the method of Powell, also recorded by Varley.[4] A standard curve was prepared over the range of 0-2 mg/100 ml for pure bilirubin; and for the liquor bilirubin, 1.0 ml of liquor, 0.2 ml of diazo reagent and 2.8 ml of sodium benzoate-urea was employed with readings taken at 530 mμ. The relationship between bilirubin and protein for 77 pairs in the 72 mothers who gave birth to babies with a positive Coombs' test or whose babies died of hemolytic disease *in utero* after the amniotic fluid was obtained showed a significant correlation ($p < 0.001$). In the presence of a dead fetus *in utero* very high values for protein and bilirubin were obtained. Wild[119] confirmed Walker's observation[108] of a fall in bilirubin concentration after the 35 weeks' gestation, but added that the protein concentration fell in a similar manner. Wild studied the electrophoretic patterns of amniotic fluid on cellulose acetate. Despite considerable variation in protein concentration, only minor variations in pattern could be shown between those fluids obtained before or after 35 weeks' gestation from fetuses who survived or died *in utero* or in the neonatal period. In sensitized pregnancies the amniotic fluid A/G ratio is normal but glycoprotein, which is normally not present in amniotic fluid, can be demonstrated.[52] Most investigators have agreed that albumin accounts for at least 50 percent of the amniotic fluid protein. However, some have not been able to find alpha-2 globulin by the conventional techniques and have assumed that amniotic fluid was a dialysate of maternal serum.[7, 78] Later Mentasti[80] by free micro-electrophoresis found results that corresponded to the changes expected in the fetus throughout gestation and not to the mother's serum. Wild's results with respect to liquor bilirubin concentration and cord bilirubin concentration tend to confirm this observation, for there is a good correlation between these two ($p < 0.001$) whereas no such relationship existed between liquor bilirubin and maternal serum bilirubin ($p > 0.5$). The protein concentration of amniotic fluid has been measured by a number of investigators[14] with values ranging from 25 to 600 mg/100 ml with an average about 350 mg/100 ml. The varying values point up the importance of describing the method, the normals for the method and the gestational age at which the samples were obtained. Walker, Fairweather and Jones[113] using the method of Folin and Ciocalteau as modified by Papadopoulos et al.[88] concluded that, although high bilirubin values tended to be associated with high protein concentrations, there were enough exceptions so that protein estimations were not as good as bilirubin values for predicting the severity of hemolytic disease in the infant. On the other hand, Cherry[33] developed a method for evaluating the amniotic fluid by determining the ratio of the $OD_{450} - OD_{600}$ to the protein concentration of the amniotic fluid. He concluded that "the use of the bilirubin/protein ratio eliminates the problem of dilution of amniotic fluid toward term and permits a diagnosis from a single specimen without knowledge of the exact stage of pregnancy." The other data referred to above would make this conclusion a little tenuous, and most investigators would prefer two amniotic fluid samples separated by a week or ten days to make any definitive diagnosis. The ratio proposed would nonetheless be of considerable help in determining the changes which might have occurred as a result of gestational age, although gestational age is of such importance in any management proposed that other confirmation must be obtained. The use of the bilirubin/protein ratio serially following intrauterine transfusion has also been proposed by Cherry to evaluate therapy, as it will gradually decrease towards normal as the infant's blood becomes entirely O-negative. The problem of heme pigments in the amniotic fluid after transfusion *in utero* has made such observations difficult to obtain, as there is frequently a seepage of blood from the peritoneal cavity of the fetus into the amniotic sac.

INTERMEDIATES OF PORPHYRIN METABOLISM

A number of precursors of heme have been described in the amniotic fluid, which include alpha-aminolevulinic acid, porphyrobilinogen, coproporphyrin I and III and protoporphyrin. Bevis[16] reported that coproporphyrin had a value of $32.7 \pm 17.7 \mu g/100$ ml which increased to a value of 220 $\mu g/100$ ml in the most severe case. The increase in coproporphyrin was mostly in isomer I, but at the highest values there were traces of III. The high value of coproporphyrin I rather than III indicates that there is some interference with the hemoglobin synthesis (I) as well as being a hemolytic process in which III would be found.[1] The other precursors have been found, for the most part, in very small amounts.[40, 104] The breakdown products found in amniotic fluid include bilirubin, bilirubin diglucuronide, urobilin, urobilinogen, oxyhemoglobin, methemoglobin, hematin, methemalbumin, hemopexin, biliverdin, mesobilirubin and porphyrins from meconium. Oxyhemoglobin, methemoglobin and methemalbumin are substances which affect the spectral absorption of amniotic fluid and contribute most to the background absorption of bilirubin at 450 mμ (Fig. 6-6).

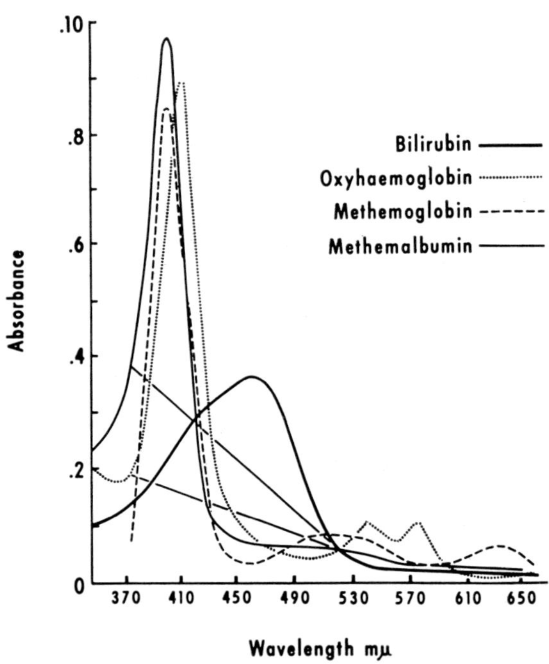

FIGURE 6-6. Spectral curves of bilirubin and other pigments. The Allen correction can be applied for background resulting from oxyhemoglobin, but calculated absorbances at 450 mμ for methemalbumin and methemoglobin are higher than actual values, but are proportional to their absorbance at 410 mμ and may be corrected for accordingly. (From Bjerre et al.[19])

Bilirubin

The degradation of hemoglobin to bilirubin can be seen in Figure 6-7. The major component of the pigments in amniotic fluid is unconjugated bilirubin.[25, 57, 73] Total bilirubin in amniotic fluid

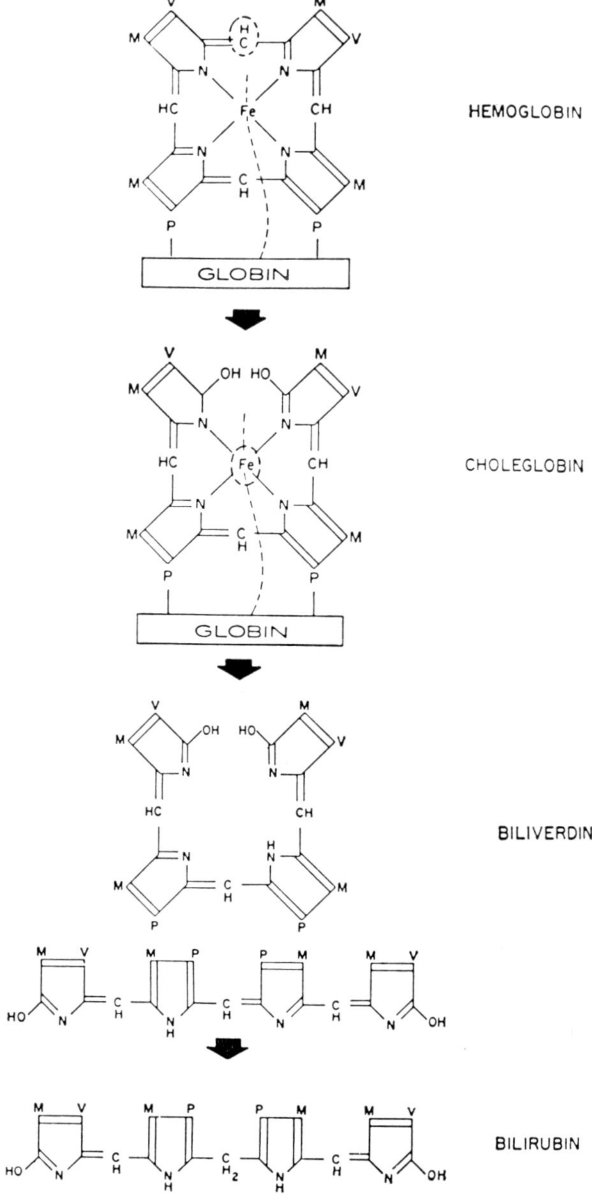

FIGURE 6-7. M = $-CH_3$ (Methyl), V = $-CH = CH_2$ (Vinyl), P = $-CH_2-CH_2-COOH$ (Proprionic Acid). The degradation of hemoglobin to bilirubin. (From Klatsin.[5])

has been estimated by the diazo method[72, 109, 115] and total and direct bilirubin was measured by Robertson in 1964.[96] Fleming and Woolf,[39] using a modified spectrophotometric method in which they determined the absorption by bilirubin itself after obtaining spectrophotometric readings at 700, 623, 576 and 462 mμ, used ratios among these readings to correct for the contribution by turbidity, methemalbumin and oxyhemoglobin. Pennington and Hall[90] further attempted to simplify and render the spectrophotometric assay of amniotic fluid more accurate by extracting the fluid with chloroform and then taking a direct reading at 450 mμ, which is corrected by an Allen correction from optical density readings taken at 420 and 480 mμ. However, it has not been definitively established whether determination of unconjugated bilirubin or the other refinements discussed above are better than the direct spectrophotometric estimation of the yellow pigment for clinical purposes (and no correction has been made for the fact that bilirubin does not obey Beer's law except when the diazo derivative is made). The variable results from different authors using different methods can be seen in Tables 6-I and 6-II.

A paradoxical increase in amniotic fluid bilirubin concentration occurs in idiopathic jaundice of pregnancy (hepatosis gravidarum)[54] and in sickle cell crisis with bilirubinemia (unpublished observation). In these situations maternal serum bilirubin increases, accompanied by a rise in cord blood bilirubin and an increase in amniotic fluid Δ OD_{450}.

TABLE 6-II

AMNIOTIC FLUID BILIRUBIN IN FOETAL HAEMOLYTIC DISEASE DETERMINED BY BIOCHEMICAL METHODS (MG/100 ML)

		Categories of Disease			
Author	*Year*	*Mild*	*Moderate*	*Severe*	*Neonatal or Foetal Death*
Kubli[59]	1966	< 0, 08	0, 08 - 0, 30	> 0, 30	
Mast[75]	1969	0, 021 - 0, 100	0, 068 - 0, 256	0, 179 - 1, 179	
Stewart[105]	1964	< 0, 035	0, 035 - 0, 060	> 0, 060	> 0, 300
Watson[116]	1965	0, 05		0, 25	0, 55

from Bartsch[5a]

Bilirubin Diglucuronide

Bilirubin diglucuronide concentration in the amniotic fluid is about 10 to 25 percent of the concentration of free bilirubin. Both free and conjugated bilirubin bind to albumin. Broderson et al.[27] have measured conjugated bilirubin diglucuronide in the amniotic fluid and theorized that bilirubin diglucuronide is in chemical equilibrium with bilirubin in the fetal liver and that both pigments are in equilibrium with the pigments in amniotic fluid. The ratio of bilirubin to bilirubin conjugate, which increases in hemolytic disease, was said to be determined by three factors: "The relative affinities of the binding to albumin, the ratio of concentrations of uridine diphosphate glucuronic acid (UDPGA) to uridine diphosphate (UDP) in the liver and the standard free energy of conjugation. The slow glycogen synthesis in the fetal liver may be responsible for a high ratio of UDPGA to UDP and hence for a high proportion of conjugated bilirubin in amniotic fluid." This is an alternate hypothesis for bilirubinemia to that hypothesis usually accepted of low transferase activity and impaired hepatic excretion before and after birth.

Urobilin; Urobilinogen

Urobilinogen has been found in a concentration of 1.79 ± 0.32 mg/100 ml in normal amniotic fluid.[16] This value was shown to fall to low values in nine stillbirths (0.55 ± 0.47 mg/100 ml).[14] Urobilin was described[121] as reaching the fetus from the maternal circulation and its drop in kernicterus made it unlikely that it would appear in the liquor amnii.[16] Although urobilinogen is usually formed from bilirubin by the action of intestinal flora, it would be expected that the fetus would have none as the fetal gut is sterile. Urobilin IXA (mesobilene-b) is said to be produced extraenterally and may be confused with urobilinogen, but none was found. The presence of and site of production of urobilinogen in the fetus is still uncertain (Fig. 6-8).

Oxyhemoglobin, Methemoglobin

The difference between the observed icterus index and that expected from the bilirubin concentration present was first thought

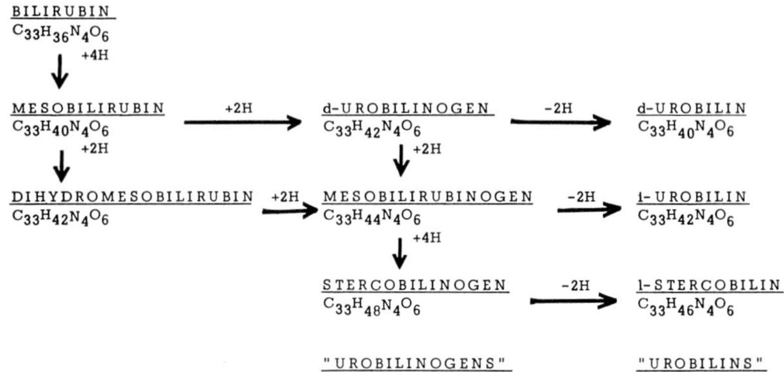

FIGURE 6-8. Conversion of bilirubin to urobilinogen. (From Klatsin.[5])

to be mesobilifuscin but turned out to be oxyhemoglobin which absorbs light, at 415, 540 and 575 mμ. Treatment of amniotic fluid with a reducing agent alters the bands to 430 and 555 mμ, and with alkaline pyridine plus sodium hydrosulfite (expected to reduce methemoglobin) sharp bands appear at 526 and 557 mμ. Hemoglobin has a broad absorption maximum near 559 mμ and a β-band of 528 mμ when heme is combined with denatured globin. The absorption of coproporphyrin in hydrochloric acid has a band near 400 mμ, which is characteristic for the porphin ring and is noted for all porphyrins regardless of their side chain and is termed the Soret band. Methemoglobin has an absorption at 634 mμ and probably occurs in very small amounts similar to the ratio in blood of less than 2 percent. Oxyhemoglobin may, in some cases following a blood tap, be present in sufficient concentration to affect the spectrophotometric evaluation of amniotic fluid for two or more weeks.

Hematin

Hematin is the iron-porphyrin compound which corresponds to methemoglobin and also is called ferric protoporphyrin. Its absorption maximum is approximately 585 mμ at pH 10. The ferri heme proteins undergo further oxidation with the formation of biliverdin. Methemoglobin oxidation following similar oxidation gives rise to choleglobin, which is one of the intermediate degradation products of hemoglobin to bilirubin (Fig. 6-7).

Methemalbumin and Hemopexin

Bevis[17] made an observation that methemalbumin appeared in high concentration in four cases of fetal death *in utero*. In peripheral blood the presence of methemalbumin is the result of recent hemolysis as it is rapidly cleared under ordinary circumstances. When it is present in amniotic fluid it may mean either an accumulation of methemalbumin in the fetal blood, which has not been cleared through the placenta and is transferred into the amniotic fluid, or the presence of excess hemoglobin breakdown pigments in the liquor as a result of intra-amniotic bleeding with a failure to metabolize the pigments to bilirubin. Apparently a poor prognostic sign when seen on spectrophotometric assay (Fig. 6-6), it must be studied further in order to completely understand the specific implications of its presence. Halitsky, Krumholz and Wiener[47] studied two hydropic infants who underwent intrauterine transfusion. They examined amniotic fluid, ascitic fluid, cord serum and first voided urine for methemalbumin (by spectrophotometric scan and Schumm's test). There was no methemalbumin in the amniotic fluid although it was present in ascitic fluid, in cord serum (in spite of three intrauterine transfusions) and in first voided urine. It is not clear whether methemalbumin is transferred through the placenta to the mother, and thus does not appear in the amniotic fluid except in cases of fetal death, or whether the previously noted hypotheses are possible.

Hemopexin is a serum glycoprotein that binds heme with a greater affinity than albumin. Hemopexin concentrations decrease as plasma heme levels rise. It has been suggested that heme as well as bilirubin may be toxic in erythroblastosis fetalis. Whether the origin of amniotic fluid hemopexin is maternal or fetal is not known. The hemopexin albumin ratio rises as gestation increases unless hemolysis is present. It has been shown that the hemopexin albumin ratio falls, reflecting the severity of the disease in the affected infant even when the spectrophotometric assay (ΔOD_{450}) may not.[84]

Biliverdin mesobilirubin and porphyrins from meconium have also been identified in amniotic fluid but in small amounts. Biliverdin is present in concentrations as low as 0-1 mg/100 ml in the absence of meconium.

Hormones

Human chorionic gonadotrophin (HCG) concentration in the amniotic fluid generally parallels that in blood or urine with a peak at 13 weeks.[12] In cases of severe erythroblastosis there is a significant elevation in amniotic fluid concentration of HCG, and the fetal cord concentration is also increased, but the increase is not significant.[13]

Whereas maternal urinary and serum concentrations of estriol do not reflect the severity of fetal disease in Rh-sensitized pregnancies,[56] estriol levels in amniotic fluid closely parallel the hemolytic process in the fetus.[102]

Additional Factors

Amniotic fluid osmolality undergoes a linear decline with increasing gestation in normal pregnancy, from a mean of about 268 at 24 weeks to 252 mOsm/kg at 40 weeks' gestation. Changes in amniotic fluid osmolality have been observed to be a more sensitive index of fetal condition than changes in bilirubin concentration.[30] Continued rise in osmolality of amniotic fluid under these conditions, rather than the normal decline, carries a poor prognosis for the fetus.

Rh-D antibody titers in amniotic fluid have also been measured[107] and found to be a reliable index of the severity of hemolytic disease in the newborn. The management of Rh-sensitized cases has not yet been carried out using such titers as an indication for induction or intrauterine transfusion. The criticism that has been levelled at the imprecision of titers in maternal serum could also be made for amniotic fluid.

Erythroblastosis can occur in relation to factors other than Rh. Those antibodies which stimulate a γ G (IgG) response are: D, c, E, K, S, Fy^a and JK^a. M, N, P, Le^a and Le^b evoke a γ M (IgM) response and are unlikely to result in erythroblastosis. The use of amniocentesis in a patient sensitized to Kell has been reported.[46] The management was successful based on the spectrophotometric assay of the amniotic fluid.

PRACTICAL COMMENTS ON SPECTROPHOTOMETRIC METHODS

The optical density "peak" at 450 mμ in normal amniotic fluid has a maximum (Δ OD_{450}) value between 18 and 20 weeks' gestation[69] of about 0.250 (Fig. 6-9). Before that time values are extremely low. The sloping lines of Liley's Zones I, II and III cannot be extrapolated back further than 28 weeks' gestation. Prior to 28 weeks, values of OD_{450} may be higher without indicating hemolytic disease. The data from Figure 6-9 have been extrapolated to Figure 6-10 to indicate the upper limits of OD deviation at 450 in normal amniotic fluid between 24 and 32 weeks. The connected points ending within the normal range were from one

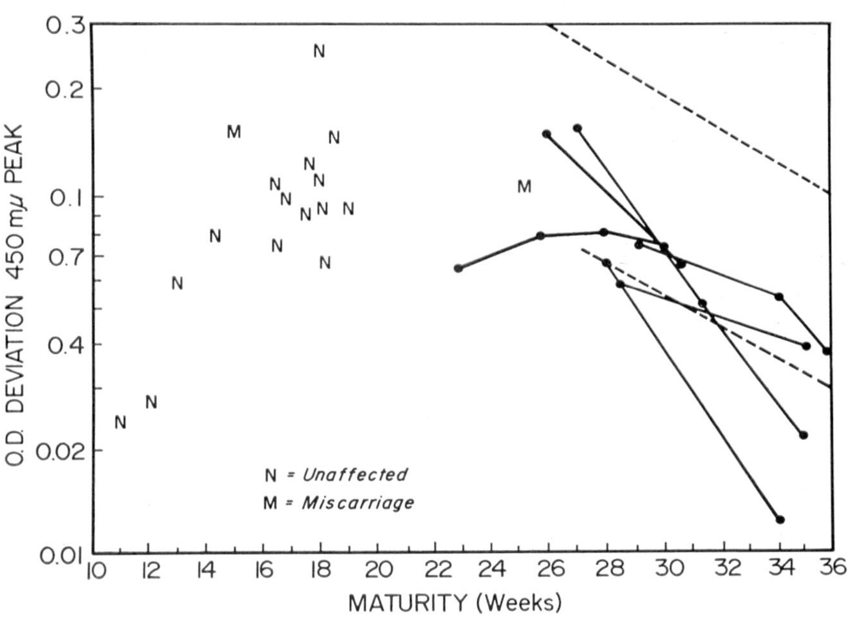

FIGURE 6-9. Pigment "peaks" in normal amniotic fluid. (From Liley.[69])

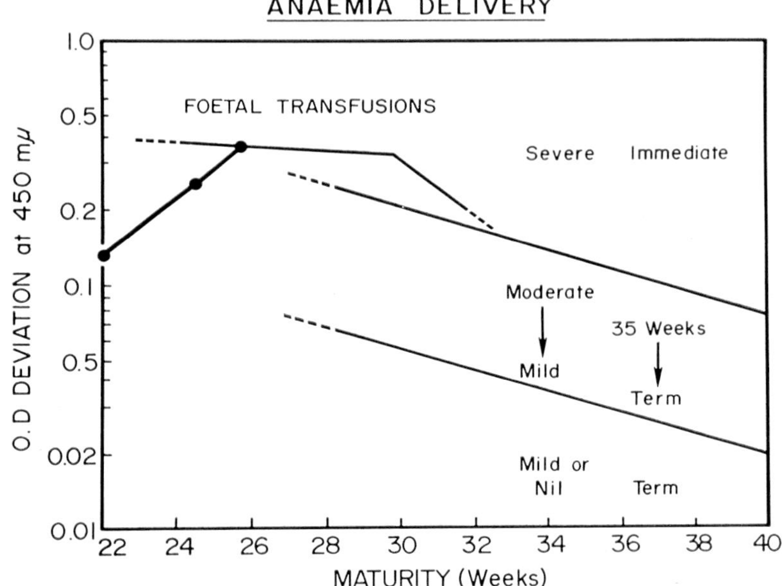

FIGURE 6-10. The significance of amniotic fluid pigment peaks in the second half of pregnancy. For the details of the three connected points, see text. (From Liley.[69])

case of Liley's in which, in spite of regular amniocentesis, the fetus died of hydrops without transfusion, which demonstrates the limitations of such "normal" ranges.

It would be helpful if agreement could be reached as to the best method to evaluate the amniotic fluid spectrophotometric curve. Figure 6-11 shows the various methods used by a number of different investigators. In this figure the base line lies between 265 mμ and 550 mμ, as Liley suggests; but others have varied it, e.g. 365 mμ and 525 mμ; 350 mμ and 550 mμ; 375 mμ and 550 mμ; 375 mμ and 525 mμ; and 365-375 mμ and 530-550 mμ (see Bartsch[5a] for details). The difference in the methods shown in the figure is based on attempts to remove background. Knox et al.[58] calculated a "liquor ratio," which is equivalent to $OD_{490-520}$, based on the assumption that the slope of the curve depends exclusively on bilirubin concentration. Bonsnes[21] corrected for hemoglobin pigment absorption (which absorbs about the same at

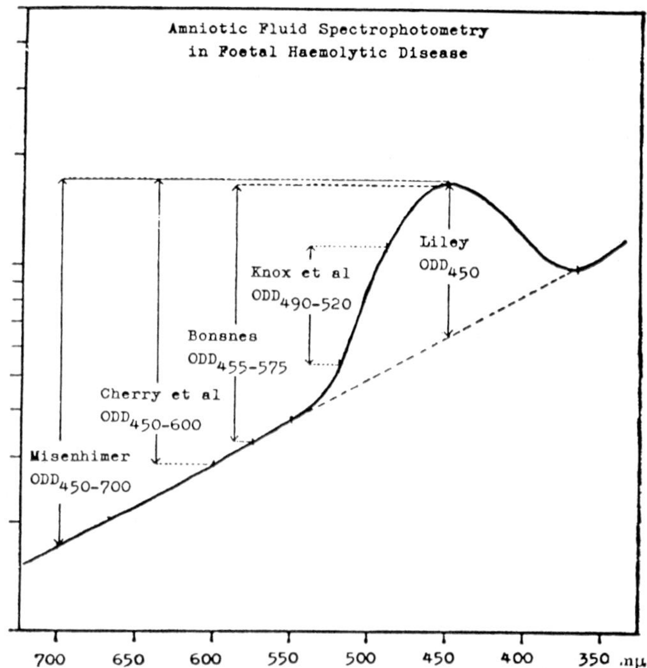

FIGURE 6-11. Measurement of bile pigment in the amniotic fluid by different spectrophotometric methods. (From Bartsch.[5])

455 mμ as 575 mμ) by his "corrected bilirubin value" $OD_{455-575}$. The others used similar "corrections."

MANAGEMENT AND PROGNOSIS BASED ON AMNIOTIC FLUID EVALUATION

The most widely used guide to management is Liley's three zones. These have only been modified by his assertion that "current criteria for foetal transfusion may be overcautious and unduly stringent."[69] This must be balanced by a caution to the inexperienced, who might overlook the necessity for establishing criteria in one's own clinic for induction and fetal transfusion, which includes the careful interpretation of amniotic fluid data and establishment of criteria for that clinic. Whitfield et al.[118] described an "action line" at which either induction or transfusion should be carried out. Although they stated that "two tests suffice to establish the further behavior of the bilirubin peak," it is not true that all third points are straight line extrapolations. The most important point from their work and others[70, 77] is that *at least* two observations must be obtained before any management is considered.

Finally, Robertson[98] has proposed a complicated and detailed chart of management which, although it is only an extension of Liley's proposed zones, may help clarify some details in the management of individual patients (Fig. 6-12).

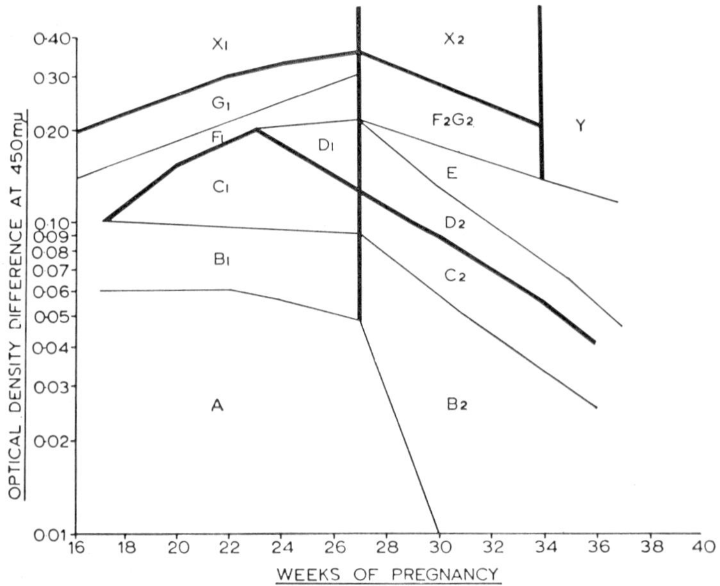

FIGURE 6-12. Graph with management zones. Zone A, repeat four weekly (2 tests) and deliver at term. Zone B_1, repeat four weekly. Zone B_2, repeat four weekly (3 tests, including Zone B_1) and deliver by term. Zone C_1, repeat three weekly. Zone C_2, repeat three weekly and delivery by 39 weeks. Zone D_1 and D_2, repeat two weekly and delivery by 38 weeks. Zone E, repeat weekly or two weekly and delivery between 36 and 38 weeks. Zone F_1, repeat two weekly. Zone G_1, repeat weekly. Zone F_2 and G_2, repeat weekly. Zone X_1 and X_2, intrauterine transfusion or operation. Zone Y, deliver immediately. (From Robertson.[98])

CONCLUSION

It appears from the data presented that (1) further investigation of the amniotic fluid content in Rh-sensitized pregnancies is important. This should include kinetic measurements where possible, (2) some agreement should be reached for standardizing the results of spectrophotometric examination of amniotic fluid, and (3) some interpretation of spectrophotometric curves of amniotic fluid into the management of the patient and her child should be agreed upon.

REFERENCES

1. Lemberg, R., and J.W. Legge: *Hematin Compounds and Bile Pigments.* New York, Interscience, 1949.
2. Queenan, J.T.: *Modern Management of the Rh Problem.* New York, Hoeber Medical Division, 1967.
3. Robertson, J.G.: Rhesus isoimmunization. In Kellar, R.J. (Ed.): *Modern Trends in Obstetrics.* New York, Appleton-Century-Crofts, 1969, pp. 202-234.
4. Varley, H.: *Practical Clinical Biochemistry.* London, Heinemann Medical Books, 1958, pp. 264, 538.
5. Klatsin, Gerald: Jaundice and other manifestations of liver disease (including tests and diagnostic features), Chapter 19. In Harrison, T.R., Raymond D. Adams, Ivan L. Bennett, Jr., William H. Resnik, George W. Thorn and M.M. Wintrobe: *Principles of Internal Medicine.* New York, McGraw-Hill, 1962.

5a. Bartsch, F.K.: Bilirubin in the amniotic fluid. *Ann. Obstet. Ginecol (Milano),* Special number, p. 73, 1970.

6. Halitsky, Victor, Burton A. Krumholz, Eugene Schwalb, and Donald S. Gromisch: The current role of intrauterine fetal transfusion in the management of erythroblastosis fetalis. *Obstet Gynecol Survey, 23:*301, 1968.
7. Abbas, T.M., and J.E. Tovey: Proteins of the liquor amnii. *Br Med J, 1:*476, 1960.
8. Allen, F.H., Jr.: Induction of labor in management of erythroblastosis fetalis. *Q Rev Pediatr 12:*1, 1957.
9. Armitage, P., and P.L. Mollison: Further analysis of controlled trials of treatment of haemolytic disease of the newborn. *J Obstet Gynaecol Br Commonw, 60:*605, 1953.
10. Baumgarten, K., and H. Frohlich: Eine einfache auswertung spektrophotometrischer fruchtwasser-kurven bei morbus haemolyticus neonatorum. *Bibl Haematol, 32:*83, 1969.

11. Beecham, Clayton T., Lyndall Molthan, Joseph Boutwell, and Charles W. Rohrbeck: Amniotic fluid studies in Rh-sensitized women. A preliminary report. *Am J Obstet Gynecol, 83:*1053, 1962.
12. Berle, P.: Der gehalt an chorialem gonadotropin im fruchtwasser wahrend normaler und pathologischer schwangerschaft. *Acta Endocrinol, 61:*369, 1969.
13. Berle, P., and H. Schultze-Mosgau: Choriales gonadotropin in mütterlichen und fetalen Blut und im Fruchtwasser bei Rh-inkompatibilität. *Arch Gynaekol, 207:*460, 1969.
14. Bevis, D.C.A.: The antenatal prediction of haemolytic disease of the newborn. *Lancet, 1:*395, 1952.
15. Bevis, D.C.A.: Composition of liquor amnii in haemolytic disease of the newborn. *Lancet, 2:*443, 1950.
16. Bevis, D.C.A.: The composition of liquor amnii in haemolytic disease of the newborn. *J Obstet Gynaecol Br Commonw, 60:*244, 1953.
17. Bevis, D.C.A.: Blood pigments in haemolytic disease of the newborn. *J Obstet Gynaecol Br Commonw, 63:*68, 1956.
18. Bevis, D.C.A.: Errors arising from amniocentesis and the origin of the liquor amnii. *J Obstet Gynaecol Br Commonw, 75:*1214, 1968.
19. Bjerre, S., C.C. Gold, R. Wilson, and T. A. Doran: Amniotic fluid spectrophotometry, urinary estrogen estimations, and intrauterine transfusion in severe Rh isoimmunization. *Am J Obstet Gynecol, 102:*275, 1968.
20. Black, J.B., G.W. Pennington, and D.W. Warrell: Clinical application of a new chemical method for the estimation of bilirubin in liquor amnii. *J Obstet Gynaecol Br Commonw, 76:*112, 1969.
21. Bonsnes, Roy W.: Model 202 analyzes bilirubin content of amniotic fluid. *Instrument News,* Perkin Elmer Corp, *16:*No. 2, 1966.
22. Bowes, Watson A., Vera E. Drose, and Paul D. Bruns: Amniocentesis and intrauterine fetal transfusion in erythroblastosis. *Am J Obstet Gynecol, 93:*822, 1965.
23. Bowman, John M., and Janet M. Pollock: Amniotic fluid spectrophotometry and early delivery in the management of erythroblastosis fetalis. *Pediatrics, 35:*815, 1965a.
24. Bowman, John M., and Janet W. Pollock: Prediction of intra-uterine death in erythroblastosis fetalis. III. Value of liquor examination. *Proc 10th Congr Int Soc Blood Transf,* Stockholm 1964, pp. 912-916, 1965b.
25. Brazie, Joseph V., Frank A. Ibbott, and Watson A. Bowes, Jr.: Identification of the pigment in amniotic fluid of erythroblastosis as bilirubin. *J Pediatr, 69:*354, 1966.
26. Brazie, J.V., W.A. Bowes, Jr., and F.A. Ibbott: An improved, rapid procedure for the determination of amniotic fluid bilirubin and its use in the prediction of the course of Rh-sensitized pregnancies. *Am J Obstet Gynecol, 104:*80, 1969.

27. Broderson, R., J. Jacobsen, H. Hertz, H. Rebbe, and B. Sorensen: Bilirubin conjugation in the human fetus. *Scand J Clin Lab Invest, 20:*41, 1967.
28. Campbell, Colin, Robert B. Jaffe, and Bruce A. Work: Statistical standardization of amniocentesis data in erythroblastosis fetalis. *Am J Obstet Gynecol, 104:*556, 1969.
29. Cary, Wilfred: Amniocentesis in haemolytic disease of the new-born. *Med J Aust, 47:*778, 1960.
30. Cassady, G., and R. Barnett: Amniotic fluid electrolytes and perinatal outcome. *Biol Neonate, 13:*155, 1968.
31. Cassady, G., and R. Barnett: Acid-base and gas tension studies of the amniotic fluid in human gestation. *Biol Neonate, 14:*251, 1969.
32. Cherry, Sheldon H.: The clinical use of amniocentesis and amniotic fluid analysis in obstetrics. *Bull Sloane Hosp Women, 13:*81, 1967.
33. Cherry, Sheldon H., and Richard E. Rosenfield: Erythroblastosis fetalis with amniotic fluid studies and intra-uterine fetal transfusions. Clinical evaluation and management. *NY State J Med, 67:*403, 1967.
34. Conradie, J.D.: The effect of millipore filtration on four spectrophotometric methods of bilirubin determination in amniotic fluid. *Clin Chim Acta, 25:*205, 1969.
35. Creasman, W.T., R.A. Lawrence, and H.A. Thiede: Fetal complications of amniocentesis. *JAMA, 204:*949, 1968.
36. Droegemueller, W., C. Jackson, E.L. Makowski, and F.C. Battaglia: Amniotic fluid examination as an aid in the assessment of gestational age. *Am J Obstet Gynecol, 104:*424, 1969.
37. Fairweather, D.V.I., S. Murray, D. Parkin, and W. Walker: Possible immunological implications of amnocentesis. *Lancet, 2:*1190, 1963.
38. Fairweather, D.V.I., and W. Walker: Obstetrical considerations in the routine use of amniocentesis in immunized Rh negative women. *J Obstet Gynaecol Br Commonw, 71:*48, 1964.
39. Fleming, A.F., and A.J. Woolf: A spectrophotometric method for the quantitative estimation of bilirubin in liquor amnii. *Clin Chim Acta, 12:*67, 1965.
40. Fikentscher, R., M. Schmidt, W. Stich, and H. Welsch: Untersuchungen über den fetalen Hämstoffwechsel. *Dtsch Med Wochenschr, 94:* 124, 1969 .
41. Freda, Vincent J., and John G. Gorman: Antepartum management of Rh hemolytic disease. *Bull Sloane Hosp Women, 8:*147, 1962.
42. Freda, Vincent J.: Management of Rh sensitized pregnancies and the special role of spectrophotometric scanning of amniotic fluid. *Bibl Haematol, 23:*919, 1965.
43. Freda, Vincent J.: Recent obstetrical advances in the Rh problem, antepartum management, amniocentesis, and experience with hysterotomy and surgery *in utero. Bull NY Acad Med, 42:*474, 1966.

44. Gambino, S. Raymond, and Vincent J. Freda: The measurement of amniotic fluid bilirubin by the method of Jendrassik and Grof. *Am J Clin Pathol, 46:*198, 1966.

45. Gairdner, Douglas, N.R. Lawrie, and Mary Hutcheon: Liquor amnii in haemolytic disease of the newborn. *Lancet, 2:*541, 1950.

46. Gusdon, John P., Norman H. Leake, and Kenneth L. Oliver: Amniotic fluid analysis in erythroblastosis secondary to Kell immunization. *Obstet Gynecol, 33:*432, 1969.

47. Halitsky, Victor, Burton A. Krumholz, and Morris F. Wiener: The significance of methemalbumin in fetal fluids. *Obstet Gynecol, 33:*339, 1968.

48. Halitsky, Victor, and Burton A. Krumholz: Amniotic fluid analysis in erythroblastosis fetalis. I. The effect of oxyhemoglobin, methemalbumin and meconium. *Am J Obstet Gynecol, 106:*1209, 1970.

49. Halitsky, Victor, and Burton A. Krumholz: Amniotic fluid analysis in erythroblastosis fetalis. II. Quantitative bilirubin relationships. *Am J Obstet Gynecol, 106:*1214, 1970.

50. Halitsky, Victor, and Burton A. Krumholz: Amniotic fluid analysis in erythroblastosis fetalis. III. The chloroform extract and its relationship to the log ΔOD_{450}. *Am J Obstet Gynecol, 106:*1218, 1970.

51. Heirwegh, K.P.M., J.A.T.P. Meuwissen, and F.H. Jansen: On the quantitation and analysis of bile pigments in amniotic fluid. *Biol Neonate, 14:*74, 1969.

52. Heron, H.J.: The electrophoresis of proteins of amniotic fluid. *J Obstet Gynaecol Br Commonw, 73:*91, 1966.

53. Horger, E.O. III, and Donald L. Hutchinson: Diagnostic use of amniotic fluid. *J Pediatr, 75:*503, 1969.

54. Jonasson, Lars Erik, and Bengt H. Persson: Spectrophotometric screening of amniotic fluid in haemolytic disease and hepatosis gravidarum. *Acta Obstet Gynecol Scand, 47:*300, 1968.

55. Kish, M.Y., John Marko, and H. Letts: Bilirubin estimation in amniotic fluid. A comparative study of 60 cases. *Am J Obstet Gynecol, 106:*592, 1970.

56. Klopper, A., and R. Stephenson: The excretion of oestriol and of pregnanediol in pregnancy complicated by Rh immunization. *J Obstet Gynaecol Br Commonw, 73:*282, 1966.

57. Kopecky, P.: Dunnschichtcromatographische Bilirubinoidanalyse des Fruchtwassers. *Geburtshilfe Frauenheilkd, 29:*818, 1969.

58. Knox, E.G., D.V.I. Fairweather, and W. Walker: Spectrophotometric measurements on liquor amnii in relation to the severity of haemolytic disease of the newborn. *Clin Sci, 28:*147, 1965.

59. Kubli, Von F., II: Die antenatale diagnose des morbus haemolyticus. *Bibl Gynaecol Fasc, 38:*30, 1966.

60. Landsteiner, K., and A.S. Wiener: Agglutinable factor in human blood recognized by immune sera for rhesus blood. *Proc Soc Exp Biol Med, 43:*223, 1940.
61. Lathe, G.H., and C.R.J. Ruthven: Factors affecting the rate of coupling of bilirubin and conjugated bilirubin in the Van den Bergh reaction. *J Clin Pathol, 11:*155, 1958.
62. Lewis, Fraser, Harold Schulman, and T. Terry Hayashi: Spectrophotometric analysis of amniotic fluid in erythroblastosis fetalis. *JAMA, 190:* 195, 1964.
63. Liley, A.W.: The technique and complications of amniocentesis. *NZ Med J, 59:*581, 1960.
64. Liley, A.W.: Liquor amnii analysis in the management of the pregnancy complicated by rhesus sensitization. *Am J Obstet Gynecol, 82:*1359, 1961.
65. Liley, A.W.: Errors in the assessment of hemolytic disease from amniotic fluid. *Am J Obstet Gynecol, 86:*485, 1963a.
66. Liley, A.W.: Intrauterine transfusion of foetus in haemolytic disease. *Br Med J, 2:*1107, 1963b.
67. Liley, A.W.: Amniocentesis and amniography in haemolytic disease. *Obstet Gynecol Year Book*, 1964-1965.
68. Liley, A.W.: The use of amniocentesis and fetal transfusion in erythroblastosis fetalis. *Pediatrics, 35:*836, 1965.
69. Liley, A.W.: Amniotic fluid pigmentation and haemolytic disease. *Bibl Haematol, 29:*237, 1968.
70. Little, Brian, Elgin McCutcheon, and Jane F. Desforges: Amniocentesis and intrauterine transfusion in Rh-sensitized pregnancy. *N Engl J Med, 274:*332, 1966.
71. Mackay, E.V.: The management of the iso-immunized pregnant woman with particular reference to amniocentesis. *Aust NZ J Obstet Gynaecol, 1:*78, 1961.
72. Mackay, E.V., and D. Watson: The prognostic value of bilirubin levels of amniotic fluid in Rhesus iso-immunized pregnancies. *Med J Aust, 49:*942, 1962.
73. Mandelbaum, Bernard, and Abner R. Robinson: Amniotic fluid pigment in erythroblastosis fetalis. *Obstet Gynecol, 28:*118, 1966.
74. See reference 95a.
75. Mast, H.: Die prantale fruchtwasseruntersuchung als basis fur die therapie bei Rh-erythroblastose. *Bibl Haematol, 32:*66, 1969.
76. Mayer, M., P. Guevitat, P. Ducas, and S. Lewi: L'examen due liquide amniotique. Element essential du prognostic antenatal de l'erythroblastose foetale. *Presse Med, 54:*2493, 1961.
77. McCutcheon, Elgin, and Brian Little: Amniotic fluid evaluation and the management of erythroblastosis fetalis. *Am J Obstet Gynecol, 98:* 266, 1967.

78. McKay, D.G., M.V. Richardson, and A.T. Hertig: Studies of the function of the early human trophoblast. III. A study of the protein structure of mole fluid, chorionic and amniotic fluids by paper electrophoresis. *Am J Obstet Gynecol, 75:*699, 1958.
79. Mellish, P., and I.J. Wolman: Intraperitoneal blood transfusions. *Am J Med Sci, 235:*717, 1958.
80. Mentasti, P.: Il protidogramma del liquido amniotico. Valutazione con microelettroforesi libera. *Minerva Ginecol,* (Torino), *11:*547, 1959.
81. Misenhimer, Harold R.: Amniotic fluid analysis in prenatal diagnosis of erythroblastosis fetalis. *Obstet Gynecol, 23:*485, 1964.
82. Misenhimer, Harold R.: Fetal hemorrhage associated with amniocentesis. *Am J Obstet Gynecol, 94:*1133, 1966.
83. Morris, E.D., John Murray, and C.R.J. Ruthven: Liquor bilirubin levels in normal pregnancy: A basis for accurate prediction of haemolytic disease. *Br Med J, 2:*352, 1967.
84. Muller-Eberhard, Ursula, and Richard Bashore: Assessment of Rh disease by ratios of bilirubin to albumin and hemopexin to albumin in amniotic fluid. *N Engl J Med, 282:*1163, 1970.
85. Nelson, George H., and O. Eduardo Talledo: Amniotic fluid spectral analysis in the management of patients with Rhesus sensitization. *Am J Clin Pathol, 52:*363, 1969.
86. Niswander, Kenneth R., Milton C. Westphal, and Swtantarta Seekree: Amniocentesis in management of the Rh problem. *Obstet Gynecol, 30:*646, 1967.
87. Ovenstone, J.A., and Aileen F. Connon: Optical density differencing: A new method for the direct measurement of bilirubin in liquor amnii. *Clin Chim Acta, 20:*397, 1968.
88. Papadopoulos, N.M., W.C. Hess, D. O'Doherty, and J.E. McLane: A procedure for the determination of cerebrospinal fluid total protein and gamma globulin in neurologic disorders. *Clin Chem, 5:*569, 1959.
89. Peddle, Leo J.: Increase of antibody titer following amniocentesis. *Am J Obstet Gynecol, 100:*567, 1968.
90. Pennington, G.W., and R. Hall: Method for the determination of small amounts of bilirubin in liquor amnii and other body fluids. *J Clin Pathol, 19:*90, 1966.
91. Pomerance, William, Arnold Moltz, Jerzy J. Biezenski, and Lewis Wolf: Spectrophotometric analysis of amniotic fluid in Rh-negative women. *Obstet Gynecol, 31:*390, 1968.
92. Queenan, J.T.: Amniocentesis for prenatal diagnosis of erythroblastosis fetalis. *Obstet Gynecol, 25:*302, 1965.
93. Queenan, J.T., and D.W. Adams: Amnocentesis: A possible immunizing hazard. *Obstet Gynecol, 24:*530, 1964.
94. Queenan, J.T., and Emmanuel Goetschel: Amniotic fluid analysis for erythroblastosis fetalis. *Obstet Gynecol, 32:*120, 1968.

95. Reddin, P.C., and Willis E. Brown: Studies on the amniotic fluid. *South Med J, 56:*287, 1963.
95a. Reil, B., G. Schellong, and H. Mast: Bestimmung der Bilirubinkonzentration im Fruchtwasser bei Rh Inkompatibilitat. *Dtsch Med Wochenschr, 94:*2602, 1969.
96. Robertson, John G.: Examination of amniotic fluid in rhesus isoimmunization. *Br Med J, 2:*147, 1964.
97. Robertson, John G.: Evaluation of the reported methods of interpreting spectrophotometric tracings of amniotic fluid in rhesus iso-immunization. *Am J Obstet Gynecol, 95:*120, 1966.
98. Robertson, John G.: Management of patients with Rh isoimmunization based on amniotic fluid examination. *Am J Obstet Gynecol, 103:*713, 1969.
99. Rosenfield, R.E., et al.: Assay of prenatal Rh antibodies to determine the need for amniotic fluid studies. *Proc, 11th Congr Int Soc Blood Transf,* Sydney, Australia, August 24 to 26, 1966.
100. Rosenfield, R.E., I.O. Szymanski, and S. Kochwa: Immunochemical studies of the Rh system: III. Quantitative hemagglutination that is relatively independent of source of Rh antigens and antibodies. *Symp Quant Biol, 29:*427, 1964.
101. Schindler, Adolf E., and V. Ratanasopa: Profile of steroid in amniotic fluid of normal and complicated pregnancies. *Acta Endocrinol, 59:*239, 1968.
102. Schindler, A.E., V. Ratanasopa, T.Y. Lee, and W.L. Herrmann: Estriol and Rh isoimmunization: A new approach to the management of severely affected pregnancies. *Obstet Gynecol, 29:*625, 1967.
103. Schmidt, M., R. Fikentscher, W. Stich, and H. Welsch: Die biochemische analyse der fruchtwasserabsorptions-bande beim morbus haemolyticus. *Bibl Haematol, 32:*78, 1969.
104. Schmidt, M., R. Fikentscher, H. Welsch, and W. Stich: Biochemische analyse der Aufbau- und Abbauprodukte des Hämoglobins, insbesondere des Bilirubins in menschlichen Fruchtwasser. *Second Internat Symposium on Foetomaternal Incompatibility, 1968.* (Bruxelles).
105. Stewart, A.G., and W. C. Taylor: Amniotic fluid analysis as an aid to the ante-partum diagnosis of haemolytic disease. *J Obstet Gynaecol Br Commonw, 71:*604, 1964.
106. Stewart, A.G., W.C. Taylor, and R.P. Beck: Amniotic fluid bilirubin levels and the Rh-isoimmunized mother. *Am J Obstet Gynecol, 97:*338, 1967.
107. Usategui-Gomez, Magdalena, Susan B. Stearns, and Helene Toolan: Rh-D antibody titer in amniotic fluids. *Am J Obstet Gynecol, 105:*1238, 1969.
108. Walker, A.H.C.: Liquor amnii studies in the prediction of haemolytic disease of the newborn. *Br Med J, 2:*376, 1957.

109. Walker, A.H.C., and R.F. Jennison: Antenatal prediction of haemolytic disease of newborn. *Br Med J, 2:*1151, 1962.
110. Walker, William: The management of rhesus iso-immunization. *J Obstet Gynaecol Br Commonw, 75:*1207, 1968.
111. Walker, W.: Role of liquor examination. *Br Med J, 1:*220, 1970.
112. Walker, W., and M.I. Ellis: Intrauterine transfusion. *Br Med J, 1:*223, 1970.
113. Walker, W., D.V.I. Fairweather, and P. Jones: Examination of liquor amnii as a method of predicting severity of haemolytic disease of newborn. *Br Med J, 2:*141, 1964.
114. Walker, W., M.J. Landon, and A. Oxley: Protein content of liquor amnii in prediction of severity of haemolytic disease of newborn. *Br Med J, 1:*605, 1969.
115. Watson, D.: The amniotic fluid bile pigments. *Proc Assoc Clin Biochem, 2:*90, 1962.
116. Watson, D., E.V. Mackay, and W. Trevella: Amniotic fluid analysis and foetal erythroblastosis. *Clin Chim Acta, 12:*500, 1965.
117. White, D., G.A. Hardar, and J.G. Reinhold: Spectrophotometric measurement of bilirubin concentrations in the serum of the newborn by the use of a microcapillary method. *Clin Chem, 4:*211, 1958.
118. Whitfield, C.R., R.A. Neely, and M.E. Telford: Amniotic fluid analysis in rhesus iso-immunization. *J Obstet Gynaecol Br Commonw, 75:*121, 1968.
119. Wild, A.E.: The association between protein and bilirubin in liquor amnii. *Clin Sci, 21:*221, 1961.
120. Willis, Charles E., and Willard R. Faulkner: Nature of the yellow pigment in amniotic fluid of mothers with Rh sensitization. (Abstracts from Scientific Sessions, Am Assoc Clin Chem 17th Nat Mtg, Chicago, 1965) *Clin Chem, 11:*814, 1965.
121. Wintermitz, M.: Urobilin in new-born; origin of urobilin. *Klin Wochenschr, 5:*988, 1926.
122. Zipursky, A., J. Pollock, B. Chown, and L.G. Israels: Transplacental foetal haemorrhage after placental injury during delivery and amniocentesis. *Lancet, 2:*493, 1963.

Chapter 7

THE FETAL PRESSURE ENVIRONMENT

Charles H. Hendricks

For nearly 100 years direct and indirect measurements of intrauterine pressures have been made. The studies have been done in response to man's curiosity as to how the uterus works during pregnancy, labor, postpartum and in the nonpregnant state. The credit for the first systematic demonstration of intrauterine pressures during pregnancies belongs to Schatz.[1]

Schatz introduced a fluid-filled bag into the uterine cavity in front of the membranes, although in some cases the membranes were inadvertently ruptured, and he then made recordings from within the amniotic cavity. With the simplest equipment, Schatz managed to demonstrate the shape of effective uterine contractions during labor, estimate their intensity, show the increase in pressure induced by voluntary bearing down and the alterations in contractility induced by change in the patient's position. His basic conclusions have never been challenged. His work was so good that some of his illustrations remained in standard textbooks for three quarters of a century.

Since the time of Schatz, dozens of modifications have been utilized by literally thousands of different workers in the recording of uterine contractile activity. It is manifestively impossible to summarize even briefly the rich literature on this subject, and only a few of these publications may be cited in this short chapter. The reader who wishes more historical detail would do well to consult the authoritative review by Reynolds, Harris and Kaiser.[2]

Dodek appears to have published the first recording of uterine contractility in labor done in the United States.[3] He prepared a simple pneumatic tambour which was strapped over the abdomen of the pregnant uterus. Increases in uterine contractility were indicated by increased tension upon the pressure system. Dodek described and portrayed the changes in normal labor and the effects of various anesthetic agents. His method was subsequently used extensively by Professor Chassir Moir[4] and by Mosteyn Embrey at Oxford in their important studies on uterine pharmacology. Subsequently, Embrey developed his own external recorder which utilizes a fluid-filled system for pressure transmittal.[5]

From 1937 to 1941, Fenning,[6-8] working with two different types of external recorders, produced beautiful records of prelabor, normal labor and abnormal labor. He laid the groundwork for mathematically assessing the quality of uterine contractility.

In 1949, Reynolds and his co-workers[9] reported the development of a multichannel strain-gage tokodynamometer which would permit external recording over different parts of the uterus simultaneously during contractions. Subsequently, Reynolds combined his efforts[10] with those of Caldeyro and Alvarez in Montevideo who had begun to make intrauterine pressure recordings in 1948.

Several other methods for recording intrauterine pressures have been described as follows: (1) open-end fluid-filled catheters inserted into the uterus,[11] (2) catheters placed into the umbilical vein after delivery of the fetus but before delivery of the placenta,[4] (3) the granular carbon microphone, used extensively in Scandinavia by Karlson,[12] and (4) telemetry from miniaturized pressure-sensitive intrauterine radio transmitters.[13] Some of the external records which have been used most extensively are the Lorand tocograph,[14] the Smythe guard-ring tocograph,[15] and the Embrey multichannel recorder.[5] Efforts to estimate uterine activity by electrohysterographic techniques have been increasingly successful, but it has not been possible to quantitatively relate electrical activity to intrauterine pressure.[16]

INTRAUTERINE PRESSURE VS. AMNIOTIC FLUID PRESSURE

Schatz identified most of the physiologic characteristics of uterine action during labor by inserting a fluid-filled bag into the extraovular space. Only on occasions, when the membranes ruptured inadvertently, did he make a recording from within the amniotic fluid cavity. Nevertheless, it has recently become customary to speak of uterine contractions only in terms of changes in the amniotic fluid pressure, which explains why this chapter is included in a book on amniotic fluid. The popularization of the term "amniotic fluid pressure" is due to the fact that Alvarez and Caldeyro-Barcia, who used that designation for the pressures they were recording in their classic work beginning in 1948,[11] have exerted such great influence upon the subsequent development of the field of uterine physiology that the term "amniotic fluid pressure" is often used when the speaker actually is referring to "intrauterine pressure."

The fact of the matter is that the amniotic fluid can claim no unique pressure of its own, since it must share its pressure environment with all the other uterine contents, including the intervillous space,[17] the extraovular space and the deep decidua. No matter in which one of these spaces one places a catheter, any recorded rise in pressure represents simply the resultant of all contractile activity being expressed upon the uterine contents at any given moment. This is because the uterus is essentially a fluid-filled vessel, and it is impossible to increase pressure in one area by uterine contractions without increasing pressure almost simultaneously and equally throughout the cavity of the uterus. Figure 7-1 illustrates this point. The top line is a tracing made from the intervillous space while the middle line tracing is recorded from the amniotic fluid. In the bottom line the two tracings are superimposed and one can see they are essentially identical. In like manner, it has been shown that the pressure in the deep decidua and also in the deepest layers of the myometrium correspond very closely to the amniotic fluid pressure.[18]

THE SIGNIFICANCE OF INTRAUTERINE PRESSURE TO THE FETUS

It is indeed fortunate for the fetus that the intrauterine pressure follows the simplest laws of hydrodynamics. If this were not the case and there was a great discrepancy between amniotic fluid pressure and the intervillous space pressure, the fetus would almost certainly be in difficulty. If during the contraction the amniotic fluid pressure rose but the intervillous space pressure remained unchanged, the fetus would tend to pump a large

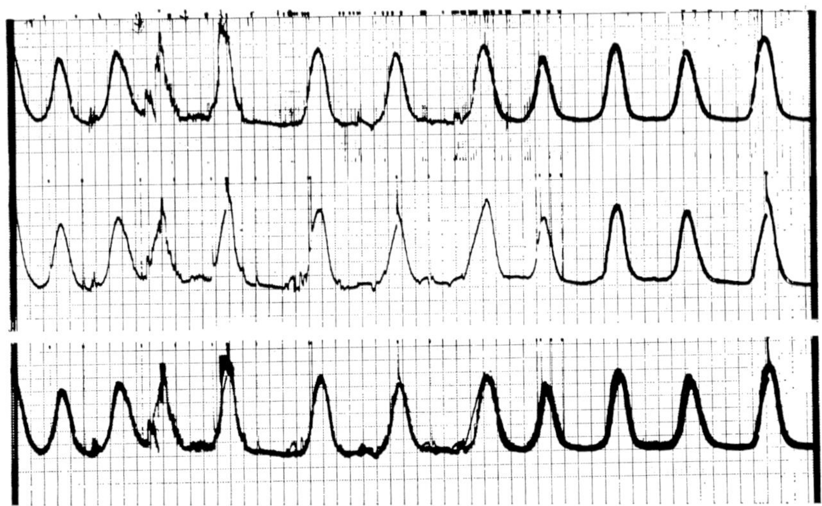

FIGURE 7-1. Superimposing the top tracing (made from the intervillous space) over the middle tracing (made from the amniotic fluid cavity) shows (lower line) that the pressure curves are virtually identical.

proportion of its blood supply into the fetal placental circulation and each contraction cycle would require major hemodynamic adjustments on the part of the fetus. On the other hand, if, during a contraction cycle, the intervillous fluid pressure rose substantially more than that of the amniotic fluid, there would be a tendency for the fetus to receive an extra large portion of the placental blood volume. This again would call for a major cardiovascular readjustment with each contraction cycle.

The uniform pressure environment permits the fetus to function without difficulty or unusual challenge. It maintains its own blood pressure, for example, in relationship to its own pressure environment as might be anticipated. Reynolds, Paul and Hugget[19] demonstrated that the fetal blood pressure rises during a uterine contraction in approximately the same amount as does the intrauterine pressure, which is as one would predict it should do.

In simple environmental pressure terms, the effect of a hard uterine contraction upon the fetus does not appear to be excessive. Consider, for example, that a very intense contraction during active labor might develop 76 mm Hg intrauterine pressure or one-tenth of an atmosphere. This is about the amount of increased pressure that would be exerted upon a person who was immersed in approximately three feet of water. Thus, one might envision the effect of uterine contractions of active labor upon the fetus as a series of slow dives to a maximum of three feet in a swimming pool approximately once every two minutes, with the intervening time being spent gliding back from that depth toward the surface as the uterus enters its relaxation phase.

During active labor, the pressure between the presenting part of the fetus and the lower portion of the uterus may be substantially greater than that of the intrauterine pressure per se, because of the direct pressure which is brought to bear as the contracting uterus pulls its lower portion up tightly around the presenting part.[20] If this process goes on for a long enough period of time, the lowermost portion of the cervix acts as a constricting band around the fetal head and the caput that forms does so because the cervix acts in a manner similar to the application of a tourniquet around an extremity.

TECHNIQUE OF RECORDING

For the past twelve years, we have recorded uterine activity from any available space within the uterine cavity, whether it be amniotic fluid, intervillous space or the extraovular space. Ordinarily open-end catheters filled with heparinized saline are introduced transabdominally to the recording site although on occasion we introduce catheters transvaginally. By this method, we can record the tonus (resting pressure between contractions) either directly with a water manometer or by arbitrarily setting the zero point in the recording system just at the height of the symphysis pubis. The tonus during pregnancy usually ranges from 4 to 10 mm Hg, occasionally rising somewhat higher during very active labor. One can also record intensity, frequency, form and pattern of uterine contractions.

PRESSURE CHANGES DURING LABOR

Before labor becomes well established, there may be several types of prelabor contractions, as shown in Figures 7-2 and 7-3. The waves are Braxton Hicks contractions. These are easily palpable by the physician, may be felt by the patient and may appear identical to those occurring in active labor except for the fact that they do not appear often enough to produce actual labor. The very small and frequent waves interspersed between the Braxton Hicks contractions are believed to represent activity of various portions of the myometrium contracting independently of the other regions. When active labor begins, this regional activity disappears.

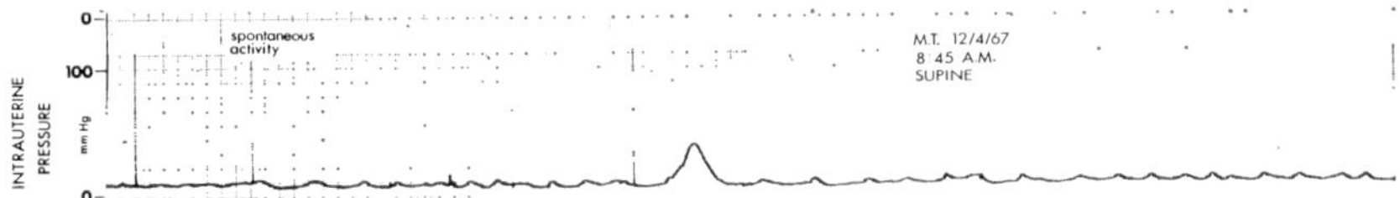

FIGURE 7-2. Prelabor. A single Braxton Hicks contraction took place during a half-hour period. The small, frequent waves represent regional contractility.

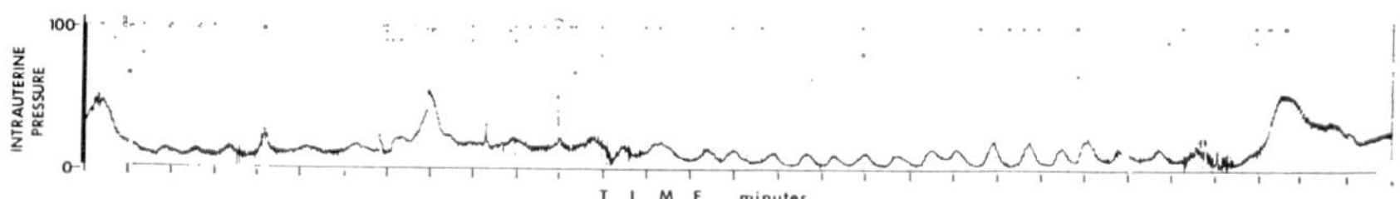

FIGURE 7-3. Prelabor. The Braxton Hicks contractions are occurring more often than was the case in Figure 2, and the regional activity waves are unusually large.

The contractions of normal labor during the active phase usually range between 35 and 80 mm Hg. One sometimes visualizes normal active labor as consisting of regular symmetrical contractions of equal intensity and occurring at precisely regular intervals. When one records pressures during a number of labors, however, this illusion is rapidly dispelled. Figure 7-4A shows a tracing from a normal spontaneous labor. Close examination reveals some variation in both frequency and intensity even in this

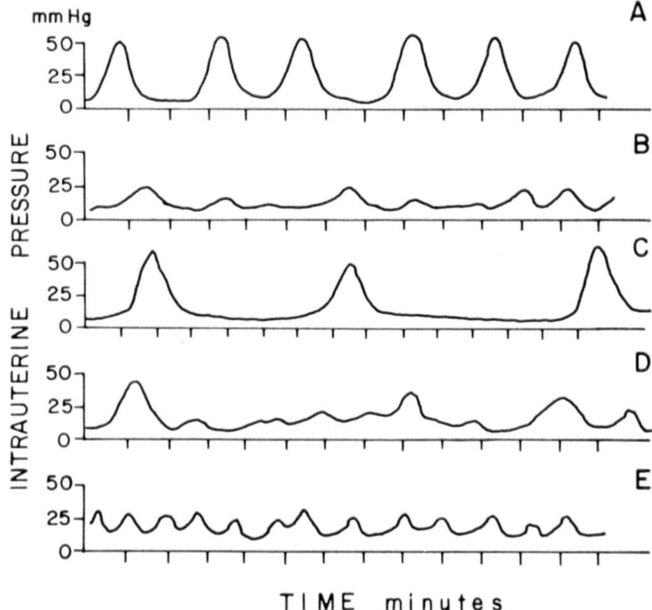

FIGURE 7-4. Various types of activity. *A,* Normal labor, typical pattern. *B,* Insufficient intensity and excessive frequency of contractions, plus some irregularity in form. *C,* Adequate contractions but insufficient frequency. *D,* Uterine incoordination. *E,* Hypercontractility of primary uterine inertia.

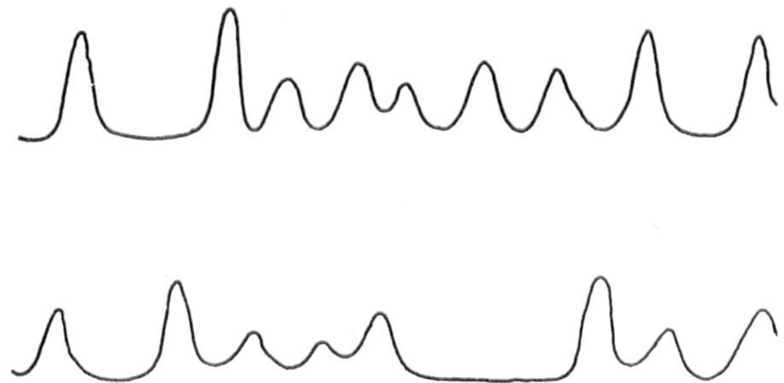

FIGURE 7-5. Bizarre contractility patterns observed during a normal spontaneous labor.

unusually uniform record. Figures 7-5–7-7 are tracings made during other normal spontaneous labors, and they show the extreme amount of variability which may occur from time to time in the course of a labor.

The effect of changing the patient's posture is shown in Figure 7-6 where at the arrow the patient turned from the supine to the lateral position. Immediately following this posture change, the pattern changed from very weak and frequent contractions to regular labor-like contractions appearing at longer intervals.

As might be anticipated, if one were to judge only from the observed contractility pattern, the dividing line between normal and abnormal labor is seldom a distinct one. Figure 7-4B shows contractions of subnormal intensity but with a frequency greater than needed for optimal performance. One would not anticipate any active progress in labor from such a pattern. In Figure 7-4C, the contractions are normal but too infrequent for labor to be efficient. Nevertheless, a certain number of patients experience what are otherwise perfectly normal labors with contractions occurring no more than every 5 to 7 minutes. Figure 7-4D is a tracing of incoordinate uterine activity which appeared after labor had begun normally. This was corrected by turning the patient to her side and instituting an oxytocin infusion at 2 mU/min. Figure 7-4E shows the hypercontractility pattern occasionally seen in primary uterine inertia.

Figure 7-8 shows the markedly dysrhythmic pattern which appeared in an obstructed labor that finally had to be terminated

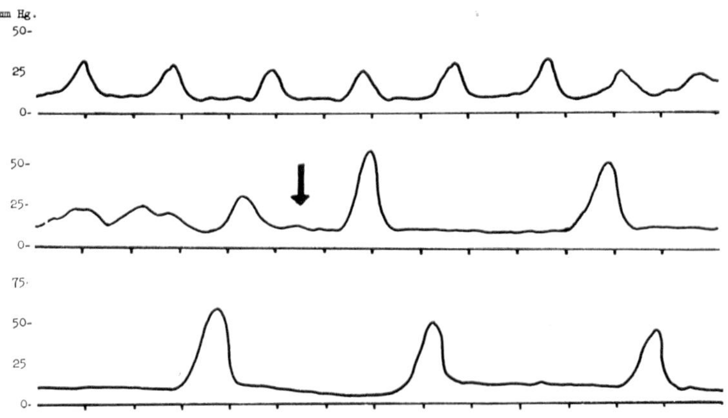

FIGURE 7-6. Early spontaneous labor. At arrow, the woman turned from the supine to the lateral position.

by cesarean section. There is no evidence, however, that this pattern is characteristic of obstructed labors because the contraction pattern in the great majority of such labors appears to be within normal limits. Furthermore, the contractility pattern of this obstructed labor does not appear particularly more bizarre than do the highly unusual patterns from normal labors shown in Figures 7-5 and 7-7.

The uterus that is overdistended tends to have contractions of less intensity than those of a normal size uterus. There is a simple explanation for this. When all the myometrial units are contracting around a relatively large intrauterine volume, the amount of observed pressure rise is less than it would be if the uterine volume had been normal. A good example of this phenomenon is a twin pregnancy where normal labor may occur with contractions of only 25 to 35 mm Hg.

In very premature labor, the intrauterine volume may be substantially less than it would have been at term. The uterine contractions often exhibit much greater intensity than would be the case at term because the intrauterine pressure appears to be inversely related to the size of the intrauterine volume about which the myometrial units are contracting.

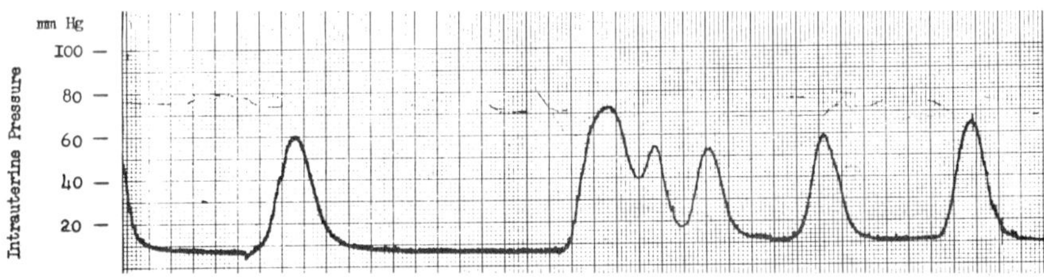

FIGURE 7-7. Unusual grouping of contractions observed in an otherwise normal labor.

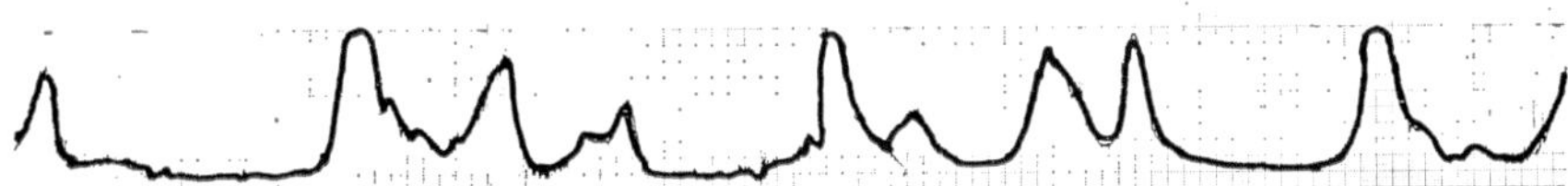

FIGURE 7-8. Abnormal contractility pattern observed in obstructed labor.

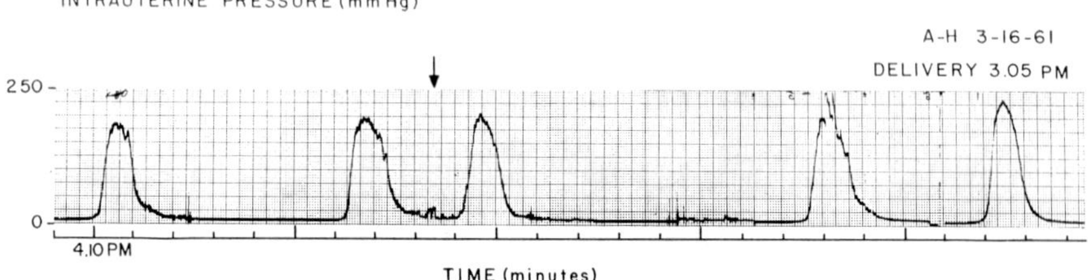

FIGURE 7-9. Uterine contractions immediately postpartum. At arrow, the placenta was delivered.

So-called hypertonus is a quite rare phenomenon in labor. It is ordinarily observed only under the following conditions:

1. Primary uterine inertia. This may be relieved by either resting the patient or turning her to the side and starting a dilute oxytocin infusion.

2. Abruptio placentae. Here the hypertonus may be very marked because of the great frequency of contractions. Thus hypercontractility is probably a more descriptive term for these cases than is the term hypertonus. Some but not all of such cases will respond to the use of oxytocin infusions.

3. Polyhydramnios. When the amniotic fluid is removed, the hypercontractility disappears.

4. Hypercontractility induced by unphysiologically large doses of oxytocin.

The uterus continues to contract spontaneously postpartum as it did antepartum. The tonus remains within the same general range as it was before labor. The contractions are substantially greater in intensity for the reason discussed above. After several hours, the contractions begin to lose their regular shape. At first, small serrations appear in the contraction patterns (Fig. 7-10). Following this the contractions become even more complex and come at increasingly infrequent intervals.

The fetus tolerates almost all aberrations and variations in uterine contractility patterns with the greatest of ease as long as the uterus relaxes reasonably well enough between contractions so that full perfusion of the placental bed can resume.

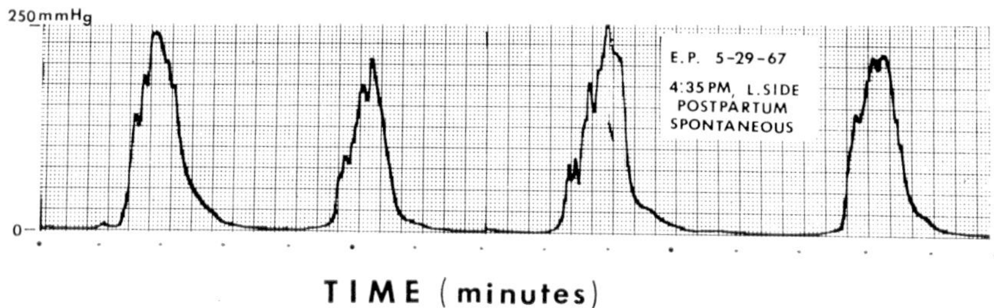

FIGURE 7-10. Contractions several hours postpartum. The process of incoordination is beginning.

Woodbury, Hamilton and Torpin,[21] in their classical work on the relationship between abdominal, uterine and arterial pressures during labor, presented evidence that during uterine contractions the effective maternal arterial pressure to the placenta might be diminished to zero. Confirmatory evidence that such a diminution does occur during the active phase of contractions has been obtained by Borell and his co-workers[22] and by Ramsey et al.[23] The arterial input to the intervillous space may be markedly reduced when the intrauterine pressure rises beyond 25 mm Hg and often during the peak of the contraction the flow is entirely cut off, thus depriving the fetus of a continuous supply of oxygen. Therefore, if these contractions come at too frequent intervals, fetal hypoxia may develop, and ultimately the fetus may exhibit the usual signs of fetal distress.

The exact point at which fetal distress will appear in response to hypercontractility is impossible to predict from the contraction pattern alone. There are, however, a few simple measures which the obstetrician may take to prevent fetal damage from hypercontractility. If contractions are coming at unusually frequent intervals, turning the patient to her left side may help reduce the frequency. If the patient is receiving an oxytocin infusion, the infusion speed should be reduced promptly. Finally, one should remember that the presence of hypercontractility may be an early indication of beginning premature separation of the placenta and that the obstetrician might wish to consider early termination of the pregnancy.

REFERENCES

1. Schatz, F.: Beitrage zur physiologischen Geburtxkunde. *Arch Gynaekol, 3:*58, 1872.
2. Reynolds, S.R.M., Harris, J.S., and Kaiser, I.H.: Clinical Measurement of Uterine Forces in Pregnancy and Labor. Springfield, Thomas, 1954, p. 5.
3. Dodek, S.M.: A new method for graphically recording the contractions of the parturient human uterus. *Surg Gynecol Obstet, 55:*45, 1932.
4. Moir, J.C.: Recording the contractions of the human pregnant and non-pregnant uterus. *Tr Edinburgh Obstet Soc, 92:*93, 1934.
5. Embrey, M.P.: A new multichannel external tocograph. *J Obstet Gynaecol Br Commonw, 62:*1, 1955.
6. Fenning, C., Davis, M.E., and Adair, F.L.: Indirect external hysterography. *Am J Obstet Gynecol, 38:*670, 1939.
7. Fenning, C.: A mechanical ink writing recorder suitable for recording uterine motility during pregnancy and labor. *Am J Obstet Gynecol, 40:*330, 1940.
8. Fenning, C.: Clinical and physiological aspects of uterine motility during pregnancy and labor. *Am J Obstet Gynecol, 43:*791, 1942.
9. Reynolds, S.R.M., Heard, O.O., Bruns, P., and Hellman, L.M.: A multi-channel strain-gage tokodynamometer: An instrument for studying patterns of uterine contractions in pregnant women. *Bull Johns Hopkins Hosp, 82:*446, 1948.
10. Caldeyro Barcia, R., Alvarez, H., and Reynolds, S.R.M.: A better understanding of uterine contractility through simultaneous recording with an internal and a seven channel external method. *Surg Gynecol Obstet, 91:*641, 1950.
11. Alvarez, H., and Caldeyro Barcia, R.: Estudios sobre la fisiología de la actividad contráctil del útero humano. Primera Communicación: Nueva técnica para registrar la actividad contráctil del útero humano grávido. *Arch Ginec y Obst Uruguay, 7:*7, 1948.
12. Karlson, S.: *A Contribution to the Methods of Recording the Motility of the Human Uterus,* Stockholm, Esselte Aktiebolag, 1944.
13. Smyth, C.N., and Wolfe, H.S.: Application of endoradiosonde or "wireless pill" to recording of uterine contractions and foetal heart sounds. *Lancet,* 1960, p. 412.
14. Lóránd, S.: (Löwi). Über einen neuen Wehenzeichnenden Apparat (Tokograph). *Zentralbl Gynaelkol, 57:*554, 1933.
15. Smyth, C.N.: The guard ring tocodynamometer. *J Obstet Gynaecol Br Commonw, 64:*59, 1957.
16. Wolfs, G., and Rottinghuis, H.: Electrical and mechanical activity of the human uterus during labour. *Arch Gynaekol, 208:*373, 1970.
17. Hendricks, C.H., Quilligan, E.J., Tyler, C., and Rucker, G.J.: Pressure relationships between the intervillous space and the amniotic fluid in human term pregnancy. *Am J Obstet Gynecol, 77:*1028, 1959.

18. Hendricks, C.H.: Amniotic fluid pressure recording. *Clin Obstet Gynecol, 9:*535, 1966.
19. Reynolds, S.R.M., Paul W.M., and Huggett, A. St. G.: Physiological study of the monkey fetus in utero: A procedure for blood recording, blood sampling, and injection of the fetus under normal conditions. *Bull Johns Hopkins Hosp, 95:*256, 1954.
20. Lindgren, L.: The importance of intra-uterine pressures and frequency of contractions during the first stage of labour. Scritti in onore del prof. Giuseppe Tesauro nel XXV anno del Suo insegnamento, Naples, Italy, 1962.
21. Woodbury, R.A., Hamilton, W.F., and Torpin, R.: The relationship between abdominal, uterine and arterial pressures during labor. *Am J Physiol, 121:*640, 1938.
22. Borell, U., Fernström, I., Ohlson, L., and Wiqvist, N.: Effect of uterine contractions on the human uteroplacental blood circulation. *Am J Obstet Gynecol, 89:*881, 1964.
23. Ramsey, E.M., Corner, G.W., Jr., Donner, M.W., and Stran, H.M.: Visualization of maternal circulation in the monkey placenta by radioangiography. Scritti in onore del prof. Giuseppe Tesauro nel XXV anno del Suo insegnamento, Naples, Italy, 1962.

Chapter 8

THE USE OF INTRA-AMNIOTIC HYPERTONIC SALINE FOR INDUCTION OF MID-TRIMESTER ABORTION

IRVIN M. CUSHNER, ALAN J. TAPPER, BRUCE THOMPSON, AND AARON S. FINK

INTRODUCTION

Interest in attaining improvements in the methodology of induced abortion has been intensified by the increasing numbers performed coincident with the very rapid changes in laws and attitudes which have occurred since 1967 in the United States and elsewhere. Actually, the use of intra-amniotic saline for inducing second trimester abortion preceded these societal changes. The procedural variations have included the use of hypertonic (50%) glucose, the transvaginal route for amniocentesis, and the use of extraovular saline.[1-10]

There have been reports of serious and fatal complications. Fatal sepsis was reported with the use of hypertonic glucose, and saline has been associated with severe hypotension, hemorrhage, cardiac arrest, renal disease, and bizarre central nervous system syndromes.[11-17]

Johnson et al.[18] reported two cases from Johns Hopkins Hospital, one of severe hypotension and one of cardiac arrest, and carried out simulation experiments on pregnant and nonpregnant dogs in which hypertonic saline was injected intravenously. The findings suggested that the clinical syndromes in these patients were probably due to intravenous injection. This eventuated in recommendations and departmental policy designed to minimize the risk of this technical accident. Thus, the procedure is delayed until 16 weeks' gestation, when the amniotic sac is more easily engaged by amniocentesis; the instillation of saline is carried out slowly and only in the presence of free-flowing amniotic fluid which is blood-free or clearing of initially present blood; and personnel are present who can monitor the vital signs during and immediately after the instillation.

The mechanism of action in this procedure is not clear. Csapo[19] has suggested, on the basis of studies in which progesterone levels and myometrial activity were measured, that saline injection into the amniotic fluid is followed by a decline in progesterone output by the placenta and then by a progressive increase in the frequency, time, and amplitude of uterine contractions. The cervix is thereby effaced and dilated (with or without rupture of the membranes) resulting in labor and evacuation of the uterus. In clinical terms, a latent period occurs between the injection and onset of symptoms when the increased myometrial activity is not yet perceptible; this is followed by abdominal (uterine) cramps, bleeding, or rupture of the membranes.

Csapo's concept is not universally accepted. Fuchs and his coworkers[20, 21, 22] were unable to discern any significant decline in progesterone output, while corroborating the progressive increase in uterine motilility to a labor-like pattern. Kerr et al.[23] studying the mechanism with hypertonic glucose, felt that evidence for trophoblastic damage was lacking and that the changes in progesterone output were not relevant.

The electrolyte changes which follow saline injection have been reviewed and studied by Anderson and Turnbull.[24] They found an immediate rise in amniotic fluid levels sodium and chloride, followed by a rapid decline over 12 hours but not to preinjection levels. Several hours after injection, while the amniotic fluid levels were falling, there was an increase in serum sodium and chloride and then an increase in urinary excretion of both. In their studies, about 60 to 70 percent of the saline injected had been excreted by the time the abortion had occurred.

At The Johns Hopkins Hospital, ten patients undergoing saline-induced abortion were studied for changes in sodium, chloride, and potassium levels in the serum, amniotic fluid, and urine. No significant changes were noted in potassium levels. Table 8-I reveals the rapid rise in amniotic fluid levels of sodium and chloride, as well as the declining levels over time. Table 8-II in-

TABLE 8-I

CHANGES IN AMNIOTIC FLUID LEVELS OF SODIUM AND CHLORIDE AFTER SALINE INJECTION

Case No.	*Pre-Injection Am. Fl. Na (mEq/liter)*	*Change (mEq)*	*Pre-Injection Am. Fl. Cl (mEq/liter)*	*Change (mEq)*	*No. Spec.*	*Time (hrs.-min.)*
1	135	1465 to 1025	111	1569 to 1109	3	0:30
2	150	1900	105	1580	2	0:01
3	133	1457	118	1252	2	0:01
4	136	1844	115	1606	2	0:01
5	134	1996	111	1772	2	0:01
6	140	1430	108	1252	2	0:01
7	134	1696	114	1712	2	0:01
8	134	1856 to 1208	113	1646 to 1065	4	0:46
9	134	2046	111	1619	2	0:01
10	136	1554 to 884	110	1310 to 760	4	0:45

TABLE 8-II

CHANGES IN SERUM LEVELS OF SODIUM AND CHLORIDE AFTER SALINE INJECTION

Case No.	*Pre-Injection Serum Na (mEq/liter)*	*Change (mEq)*	*Pre-Injection Serum Cl (mEq/liter)*	*Change (mEq)*	*No. Spec.*	*Time (hrs.-min.)*
1	138	−7 to +4	109	0 to +3	9	12:00
2	135	−2 to +2	106	0 to +3	6	10:13
3	129	0 to +9	93	+4 to +5	8	6:40
4	127	+6 to +10	107	+13 to 17	6	6:05
5	135	0 to +3	102	+5 to +7	6	8:04
6	133	0 to +4	97	0 to +5	7	7:05
7	139	−1 to +2	105	+2 to +5	8	3:40
8	136	+2 to +7	98	+4 to +13	8	5:50
9	135	0 to +5	106	−4 to +4	6	6:57
10	143	−5 to −2	107	+3 to +4	7	4:19

dicates more consistent increases in serum chloride than in sodium, both being of a relatively low order. In Table 8-III, the gradually increasing urinary excretion of both is noted.

TABLE 8-III

CHANGES IN URINARY EXCRETION OF SODIUM AND CHLORIDE AFTER SALINE INJECTION

Case No.	*Pre-Injection Urine Na (mEq/liter)*	*Change (mEq)*	*Pre-Injection Urine Cl (mEq/liter)*	*Change (mEq)*	*No. Spec.*	*Time (hrs.-min.)*
1	107	47 to 147	?	?	4	14:12
2	169	74 to 159	134	38 to 194	4	7:13
3	174	77 to 80	169	47 to 94	4	6:45
4	71	71 to 82	71	31 to 58	3	6:32
5	187	—50	177	—21	2	1:20
6	?	?	?	?	3	6:18
7	129	57 to 69	121	87 to 91	3	4:40
8	236	—36	170	52	2	6:10
9	152	121 to 248	176	87 to 107	4	6:23
10	248	122	202	101	2	5:35

The role of intra-amniotic saline which has emerged in most abortion programs is to replace abdominal hysterotomy, which previously was the only available method in patients whose pregnancy had progressed beyond 12 weeks of gestation. The frequency of its use, therefore, reflects the incidence of late reporting of unwanted pregnancies and the effects of procedural delays in providing the service. Table 8-IV reveals the number of abortions performed and the distribution by method in Maryland and at The Johns Hopkins Hospital since the enactment of a liberalizing abortion law. It can be seen that while the frequency of use of saline is declining, over one third of the patients have required it.

There have been no deaths among the saline-induced abortions performed at The Johns Hopkins Hospital through June 30, 1971. It should be noted, however, that there have been three deaths among 12,723 abortions performed in Maryland hospitals since enactment of the new abortion law. They all followed saline-induced abortion and were associated with sepsis. One of these deaths occurred five weeks after an uneventful hospital and post-

TABLE 8-IV

METHODS OF HOSPITAL-PERFORMED ABORTION IN MARYLAND AND AT THE JOHNS HOPKINS HOSPITAL

	Total Abortions	*Suction Curettage*	*Saline*	*Abdominal*	*Deaths*
Maryland					
7/1/68 to 6/30/69	2134	1015	888 (41.6%)	231	0
7/1/69 to 6/30/70	5530	2966	1972 (35.7%)	592	3
7/1/70 to 3/31/71*	5059	2944	1658 (32.8%)	457	0
TOTAL	12723	6925	4518 (35.5%)	1280	3
Johns Hopkins Hospital					
7/1/68 to 6/30/69	1178	441	617 (52.3%)	120	0
7/1/69 to 6/30/70	1630	750	685 (42.0%)	195	0
7/1/70 to 6/30/71	2408	1344	897 (37.3%)	167	0
	5216	2535	2199 (42.2%)	482	0

*As of this writing, data are not yet available for the fourth quarter of fiscal year 1970-71.

abortal course; the other two were clearly related to the procedure.

The first saline-induced abortion to be done at The Johns Hopkins Hospital was carried out in 1964. During the first five years of its use, 586 were performed (Table 8-V). These cases have been reviewed for patient characteristics, methodology, and results. This review forms the basis for the remainder of this chapter.

TABLE 8-V

SALINE-INDUCED ABORTION PERFORMED JOHNS HOPKINS HOSPITAL, 1964-1968

Year	*Number*
1964	8
1965	12
1966	44
1967	179
1968	343
	586

PATIENT CHARACTERISTICS

Almost two thirds of these patients had never before been pregnant (Table 8-VI). Of the multigravidae, 60 percent had three previous pregnancies or less, and the remainder had four or more. There was no patient whose parity was over seven.

The age distribution is seen in Table 8-VII. Eighty-six percent were under age 30; 35.5 percent were under age 20.

The distribution by marital status, as shown in Table 8-VIII, indicates that 14.8 percent had previously been married, but were not married at the time of the procedure, while 64.2 percent had never married. Thus, 79.0 percent of all patients were not married when the abortion was needed.

TABLE 8-VI

GRAVIDITY

Gravidity	*No.*	%
Unknown	11	1.9
0	373	64.7
1-7	202	33.4
	586	100.0

TABLE 8-VII

AGE

Age	*No.*	%
Unknown	3	0.5
Under 15	22	3.8
15-19	186	31.7
20-24	219	37.4
25-29	76	13.0
30-34	42	7.2
35-39	24	4.0
40+	14	2.4
	586	100.0

TABLE 8-VIII

MARITAL STATUS

Marital Status	*No.*	*%*
Unknown	16	2.7
Married	107	18.3
Never married	376	64.2
Sep. div. wid.	87	14.8
	570	100.0

In a large majority of the patients (88.4%), the procedure was done between 16 and 22 weeks following the last menstrual period. Those under 12 weeks were among the earliest cases in this series, and such patients are no longer considered candidates for the saline method (Table 8-IX).

As is the case in most hospitals performing large numbers of abortions, the most common indication for the operation was one involving psychosocial factors; these accounted for 90.5 percent of the cases. Table 8-X reveals that those done for fetal indications represented 3.6 percent, and included cases of exposure to

TABLE 8-IX

DURATION OF PREGNANCY

Pregnancy Duration (Weeks from LMP)	*No.*	*%*
Unknown	21	3.5
Under 12	8	1.4
12-15	78	13.3
16	82	14.0
17	113	19.3
18	99	16.9
19	71	12.1
20	55	9.4
21-22	39	6.7
23+	20	3.4
	586	100.0

TABLE 8-X

INDICATIONS

Indication	*No.*	%
None listed	19	3.2
Mental health	530	90.5
Fetal	20	3.4
Rape	9	1.5
Physical health	8	1.4
	586	100.0

rubella, excessive irradiation, and other adverse factors indicated by cytogenetic studies.

METHODOLOGY

Preinjection Management

Initially, patients were managed as inpatients, being admitted the day prior to injection and remaining in the hospital until after complete evacuation. More recently, however, practices have changed, and they are now admitted after the injection. A study now under way indicates that it is safe to allow the patient to leave the hospital after a suitable period of postinjection observation, to return at the onset of symptoms for uterine evacuation.

Most patients receive some form of preinjection sedation. This is usually given intravenously or intramuscularly, and it has included phenothiazine, meperidine, or a barbiturate.

Currently, amniocentesis and saline instillation are carried out in the delivery suite, which, for obvious reasons, is most unsatisfactory. In general, it can be assumed that the optimal area for abortion procedures would be one which does not include the management of obstetrical patients who are to deliver at term. The facility, however, must allow for a period of postinjection observation when the intensiveness of care would be similar to that of a partially recovered patient following abdominal surgery (e.g. postoperative recovery room or a postoperative nursing unit).

Technique

The patient is placed in the dorsal recumbent position. The anterior abdominal wall is prepared with Betadine.® The site for amniocentesis is selected about 3 to 4 cm below the palpable fundus and over an area where palpable cystic consistency would indicate underlying amniotic fluid. The site is infiltrated with 1% Xylocaine.®

The needle must be of sufficient length and bore to allow for engaging the amniotic cavity and for a free flow of amniotic fluid. Those of the type used for spinal anesthesia are satisfactory, particularly the Tuohy needle, whose blunt end and laterally located opening should minimize the risk of obstruction by fetal parts. A more recent innovation is that of replacing the needle with polyethylene tubing for the fluid withdrawal and saline instillation. Those products in which the needle is encased in a tube of polyethylene allow the needle to be withdrawn and the tube to remain, and are quite satisfactory.

Table 8-XI indicates the experience with the amniocentesis itself. It will be noted that in the great majority of cases, the amniotic cavity is engaged with a single primary attempt. "Primary" designates the first instance at which amniocentesis is accomplished, either by single or multiple attempts at entering the amniotic sac. A "secondary" attempt is carried out at a subsequent time, usually as a result of some technical difficulty during the

TABLE 8-XI

ATTEMPTS AT AMNIOCENTESIS

Number Attempts	*No.*	%
Unknown	36	6.1
1	458	78.2
2	44	7.5
3	12	2.0
4	11	1.9
5+	25	4.3
	586	100.0

primary procedure. The high proportion of single, primary tap is presumably related to duration of pregnancy and its associated fluid volume and uterine size.

The amniocentesis is followed by withdrawal of fluid or by instillation of 20% saline or both. Several techniques are used. Initially, they included a method ("in-out") in which fluid was first removed in 50 cc increments and immediately followed by the instillation of saline at the same rate. Another method ("exchange") involved alternately withdrawing and injecting in the same increments. These are the two methods presented in this 5-year report. Subsequently, other techniques have evolved. They include (1) saline injection without prior removal of fluid but allowing a free flow between syringefuls, and (2) introduction of the saline through an infusion drip with or without prior removal of fluid.

Other variants in technique have to do with the total amount of fluid removed, the total amount of saline injected, and the differences between them. Table 8-XII reveals the distribution of amounts of fluid removed and Table 8-XIII reveals that of the amounts of saline injected. Table 8-XIV displays the distribution of the differences in volumes removed and injected. These data indicate that (1) in most cases the volume removed and that injected was between 100 and 300 ml, (2) there was a tendency to remove smaller volumes and to inject larger ones, and (3) in

TABLE 8-XII

AMOUNT OF AMNIOTIC FLUID REMOVED

Amount (cc)	*No.*	*%*
Unknown	42	7.2
0-99	36	6.1
100-199	126	21.5
200-299	229	39.1
300-399	85	14.5
400+	68	11.6
	586	100.0

86 percent, the amount injected was either equal to or greater than that removed.

Among 533 cases, in which the technique used and the volume differences are both known (Table 8-XV), the data indicates an

TABLE 8-XIII

AMOUNT OF HYPERTONIC SALINE INJECTED

Amount (cc)	*No.*	*%*
Unknown	33	5.6
0-99	10	1.7
100-199	48	8.2
200-299	300	51.2
300-399	119	20.3
400+	76	13.0
	586	100.0

TABLE 8-XIV

DIFFERENCES BETWEEN AMOUNT OF FLUID REMOVED AND AMOUNT OF SALINE INJECTED

Amount Injected Minus Amount Removed (cc)	*No.*	*%*
Unknown	48	8.2
100 or more	66	11.3
75 to 99	22	3.8
50 to 74	78	13.3
25 to 49	67	11.4
1 to 24	18	3.1
0	251	42.9
—1 to 24	6	1.0
—25 to 49	12	2.0
—50 to 74	6	1.0
—75 to 99	2	0.3
—100 or more	10	1.7
	586	100.0

TABLE 8-XV

DISTRIBUTION BY METHOD OF INJECTION AND VOLUME DIFFERENCE

Volume Difference	*"In-Out"*	*"Exchange"*	*Total*
Equal	66	187	253
Injection more	181	63	244
Injection less	22	14	36
	269	264	533

"In-Out" = The removal of amniotic fluid in 50 cc increments, then followed immediately by the injection of 20% saline in 50 cc increments.

"Exchange" = Alternating the removal of 50 cc of fluid from the amniotic cavity with the injection of 50 cc of hypertonic saline.

almost equal distribution of the techniques and a greater use of overdistension with the "in-out" method.

It is our practice to observe these patients in a recovery room setting for about one hour following injection. This is particularly important for those who have received sedation, but it is equally important for the discernment of abnormal levels of pulse rate, blood pressure, and respiration, as well as the thirst and headache which might occur with significant hypernatremia. When these have occurred, they have generally been short in duration and subside spontaneously.

When fully recovered and stable, the patients are transferred to a gynecologic-obstetric nursing unit where they are allowed ambulation and a regular diet. At the onset of uterine contractions, vaginal bleeding, or rupture of membranes, they are transferred to the operative area for management of the uterine evacuation. Analgesia is used during this phase and generally consists of meperidine, with or without phenothiazine.

As regards the use of oxytocin, 83 percent of the patients received an infusion containing 10 cc of oxytocin in 1000 cc of intravenous fluid. Table 8-XVI indicates the general practice of initiating oxytocin stimulation after the onset of contractions. Those cases in which oxytocin infusion was used earlier were either those in which membranes had ruptured or in which the

TABLE 8-XVI

USE OF OXYTOCIN INFUSION

	No.	*%*
Used before onset	76	13.0
Used after onset	410	70.0
Not used	100	17.0
	586	100.0

TABLE 8-XVII

DURATION OF INTERVAL BETWEEN INJECTION AND ONSET OF ABORTION

Hours	*No.*	*%*
Unknown	44	7.5
Under 4	12	2.0
4-8	37	3.6
8-12	49	8.4
12-16	67	11.5
16-20	60	10.2
20-24	57	9.7
24-28	71	12.2
28-32	43	7.3
32-36	47	8.0
36-40	29	4.9
40+	70	12.0
	586	100.0

latent period had exceeded 18 to 24 hours. More recently, there has been increasing use of oxytocin at earlier times in the latent period in the hope of reducing it.

RESULTS

Time Intervals

Tables 8-XVII, 8-XVIII, and 8-XIX reveal the distribution of time interval groups for the intervals between injection and onset,

TABLE 8-XVIII

DURATION OF INTERVAL BETWEEN ONSET AND COMPLETION OF ABORTION

Hours	*No.*	*%*
Unknown	47	8.0
Under 3	123	21.0
3-6	131	22.4
6-9	77	13.1
9-12	67	11.4
12-15	50	8.5
15-18	29	5.0
18-21	20	3.4
21-24	17	2.9
24-36	17	2.9
36-48	3	0.5
48+	5	0.9
	539	100.0

TABLE 8-XIX

DURATION OF INTERVAL BETWEEN INJECTION AND COMPLETION OF ABORTION

Hours	*No.*	*%*
Unknown	25	4.3
Under 6	0	0.0
6-12	7	1.2
12-18	47	8.0
18-24	104	17.7
24-30	102	17.4
30-36	106	18.1
36-42	62	10.6
42-48	49	8.4
48+	84	14.3
	561	100.0

onset and evacuation, and injection and evacuation. The median case for the injection-onset interval is at 20 to 24 hours; in the onset-evacuation interval it is at 6 to 9 hours; and in the total injection-evacuation time, 30 to 36 hours. In all three groups, there are some unusually short and long time intervals recorded. Further studies are underway to seek any correlations between interval and certain features of methodology or patient characteristics.

Complications

The most common complication in this series was placental retention for more than one hour following delivery of the fetus. The incidence was 43 percent. Table 8-XX reveals that most of these cases were managed by surgical means. About half of the surgical procedures required curettage and anesthesia; the other half were removed manually from the cervix or vagina or by the use of "sponge-stick" grasping instruments without anesthesia. Thus, of the total series, 88 patients (15%) required an anesthetic procedure.

The other complications are tabulated in Table 8-XXI. The incidence of specific infection was 10.0 percent; eight additional

TABLE 8-XX

COMPLICATIONS: RETAINED PLACENTA

Retained Placenta (1 + hr.)	*No.*		
Spontaneous delivery 1-2 hr.	38		
Spontaneous delivery 2-3 hr.	16		
Spontaneous delivery 3-4 hr.	10		
Spontaneous delivery 4+ hr.	13		
Nonsurgical		77	
Manual removal	54		
Sponge-stick removal	35		
D & C alone	49		
D & C plus removal	39		
Surgical		177	
Total		254	(43.3%)

TABLE 8-XXI

OTHER COMPLICATIONS

	No.	%
Infection		
Puerperal	41	7.0
Urinary tract	10	1.7
Puerperal and urinary	2	0.3
Thrombophlebitis	6	1.0
Fever, cause?	8	1.4
Total infection	67	11.4
Shock	4	0.7
Transfusion		
500 cc	5	0.85
1000 cc	5	0.85
2000 cc	1	0.17
More than 2000 cc	3	0.51
Total transfusion	14	2.38

cases were febrile with no clinically discernible explanation. Four patients exhibited clinical shock which required either whole blood or plasma volume expander. Fourteen patients suffered sufficient blood loss to warrant blood transfusions, four of them requiring more than 1000 cc.

Technical Difficulties

Four types of technical difficulties were encountered in these patients: (1) those in which no fluid could be obtained at amniocentesis; (2) those in which fluid was initially obtained, but quickly became unobtainable due to obstruction or inadvertent removal of the needle or tubing from the amniotic cavity; (3) those in which the fluid was persistently bloody without evidence of clearing; and (4) those in which there were no clinical signs of uterine activity or membrane rupture within 24 hours after saline injection. The method by which these difficulties were managed are noted in Table 8-XXII, where it is seen that the difficulties with

TABLE 8-XXII
MANAGEMENT OF TECHNICAL DIFFICULTIES

	No.	Management		
		Secondary Attempt	Oxytocin	Hysterotomy
No fluid	19	16	1	2
Inadequate fluid	2	2	0	0
Bloody fluid	19	10	4	5
Inadequate response	102	8	88	6
Total	142	36	93	13

the fluid were rather uncommon, while inadequate response was noted in 17.4 percent of the cases. Of the total 142 cases, 129 were successfully aborted either by a secondary amniocentesis at a subsequent time or by oxytocin infusion or both. In the remaining thirteen cases, hysterotomy was deemed necessary; these represent 2.2 percent of the total series.

REFERENCES

1. Stann, O., and DeWatteville, H.: Etude experimentale sur le mecanisme d'avortement par hydramnios artificil. *Gynecol Obstet, 53:*171-187, 1954.
2. Brosset, A.: The induction of therapeutic abortion by means of a hypertonic glucose solution injected into the amniotic sac. *Acta Obstet Gynecol Scand, 37:*519, 1958.
3. Svane, H.: Interruption of pregnancy by intrauterine instillation of saline. *Dan Med Bull, 7:*51, 1960.
4. Bengtsson, L.P., and Csapo, A.I.: Oxytocin response, withdrawal and reinforcement of defense mechanism of the human uterus at midpregnancy. *Am J Obstet Gynecol, 83:*1083, 1962.
5. Amris, C.J., and Jepsen, O.B.: Intravenous infusion as a complication in therapeutic abortion by the intrauterine extraovular hypertonic saline method. *Dan Med Bull, 9:*143, 1962.
6. Jaffin, H., Kerenyi, T., and Wood, E.C.: Termination of missed abortion and the induction of labor in midtrimester pregnancy. *Am J Obstet Gynecol, 84:*602, 1962.
7. Wood, C., Booth, R.T., and Pinkerton, J.H.M.: Induction of labour by intra-amniotic injection of hypertonic glucose solution. *Br Med J, 2:* 706, 1962.

8. Sciarra, J.J., King, T.M., and Steer, C.M.: Induction of labor by the intra-amniotic instillation of hypertonic solutions. *Bull Sloane Hosp Women, 10:*48, 1964.
9. Wagatsuma, T.: Intra-amniotic injection of saline for therapeutic abortion. *Am J Obstet Gynecol, 93:*743, 1965.
10. Ruttner, B.: Termination of mid-trimester pregnancy by transvaginal intra-amniotic injection of hypertonic solution. *Obstet Gynecol, 28:*601, 1966.
11. Cameron, J.M., and Dayan, A.D.: Association of brain damage with therapeutic abortion induction by amniotic fluid replacement: report of two cases. *Br Med J, 3:*1010, 1966.
12. MacDonald, D., O'Driscoll, M.K., and Geohegan, F.J.: Intra-amniotic dextrose—a maternal death. *J Obstet Gynaecol Br Commonw, 72:*452, 1965.
13. Eisner, G.M., and Piver, J.S.: Acute renal failure after therapeutic abortion by intra-amniotic saline administration. *New Engl J Med, 279:*360, 1968.
14. Cameron, J.M., Morgan, A.G., Robinson, A.E., and Urich, H.: Brain damage following therapeutic abortion by amniotic fluid replacement: an experimental approach. *J Obstet Gynaecol Br Commonw, 76:*168, 1969.
15. Goodlin, R.C., McLennan, C.E., Choyce, J.M., Lee, R.S., and Steckler, J.E.: Therapeutic abortion with hypertonic intra-amniotic saline. A clinical experience in a combined community-university hospital. *Obstet Gynecol, 34:*1, 1969.
16. Futoran, J.M., Lowenstein, J.M., and Peacock, W.G.: Experience with intra-amniotic hypertonic saline injections: Aburel's procedure. *Am J Obstet Gynecol, 105:*191, 1969.
17. Bahary, C., Goldman, J., and Eckerling, B.: Placenta previa: a contraindication to the intrauterine injection of hypertonic saline solution. *Int Surg, 53:*304, 1970.
18. Johnson, J.W.C., Cushner, I.M., and Stephens, N.C.: Hazards of using hypertonic saline for therapeutic abortion. *Am J Obstet Gynecol, 94:* 225, 1966.
19. Csapo, A.I.: In *Yearbook of Obstetrics and Gynecology, 1966-1967,* Greenhill, J.P., (ed.), Chicago, Yearbook Medical Publishers, 1966, p. 126.
20. Fuchs, F., Fuchs, A.R., Short, R.V., and Wagner, G.: Uterine motility and concentrations of progesterone in uterine venous blood after intra-amniotic injection of hypertonic saline. *Acta Obstet Gynecol Scand, 44:*63, 1965.
21. Short, R.V., Wagner, G., Fuchs, A.R., and Fuchs, F.: Progesterone concentrations in uterine venous blood after intra-amniotic injection of hypertonic saline in midpregnancy. *Am J Obstet Gynecol, 91:*132, 1965.

22. Moller, K.J.H., Wagner, G., and Fuchs, F.: Inability of progestagens to delay abortion induced with hypertonic saline. *Am J Obstet Gynecol, 90:*694, 1964.
23. Kerr, M.G., Roy, E.J., Harkness, R.A., Short, R.V., and Baird, D.T.: Studies of the mode of action of intra-amniotic injection of hypertonic solutions in the induction of labor. *Am J Obstet Gynecol, 94:*214, 1966.
24. Anderson, A.B.M., and Turnbull, A.C.: Changes in amniotic fluid, serum, and urine following the intra-amniotic injection of hypertonic saline. *Acta Obstet Gynecol Scand, 47:*1, 1968.

INDEX

S

T

U